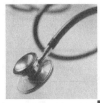
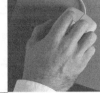

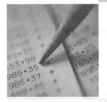

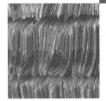

W9-AAO-743

THE BUSINESS OF MEDICINE

An Essential Guide for

Obstetrician – Gynecologists

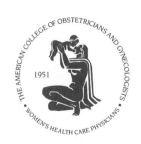

The American College of
Obstetricians and Gynecologists
Women's Health Care Physicians

The Business of Medicine: An Essential Guide for Obstetrician–Gynecologists was developed by the following staff members of the Department of Health Economics of the American College of Obstetricians and Gynecologists (ACOG):

Albert L. Strunk, JD, MD, FACOG, Vice President, Fellowship Activities
James Scroggs, Director, Department of Health Economics
Anne Diamond, Manager, Practice Management
Marian Wiseman, MA, Consultant

The American College of Obstetricians and Gynecologists would like to extend special thanks to the following individuals for their contributions and guidance:

May Hsieh Blanchard, MD
Tamara Helfer, MD, MBA
Wanjiku N. Kabiru, MD
Stephen Klasko, MD, MBA
Erica Marsh, MD
Sarah Kline, JD, ACOG Staff Attorney

Library of Congress Cataloging-in-Publication Data

The business of medicine : an essential guide for obstetrician-gynecologists / the American College of Obstetricians and Gynecologists, Women's Health Care Physicians; [developed by Albert L. Strunk, et al.].
    p. ; cm.
Includes index.
ISBN 1-932328-14-9
    1. Medicine—Practice. 2. Gynecology—Practice. 3. Obstetrics—Practice. [DNLM: 1. Obstetrics. 2. Practice Management, Medical—organization & administration. 3. Gynecology. WQ 21 B979 2005] I. Strunk, Albert L. II. American College of Obstetricians and Gynecologists.
R728.B885 2005
618'.068—dc22

                                                                    2004028927

Contents

Preface

Changes in the U.S. health care system that have taken place over the past two decades have made the health care industry subject to many of the same forces of the free market that prevail in other businesses. Although physicians may be paid through a variety of mechanisms, including self-payment made directly by patients, entitlement programs (Medicare, Medicaid, and Tricare), traditional indemnity plans, and managed health care plans, it is "the managed care revolution" that has radically altered the health care system of the United States. The primary factor fueling the move toward managed care is the increasing cost of health care, which makes up an ever-growing portion (approximately 15%) of the nation's gross national product. Nearly two thirds of Americans younger than 65 years receive health insurance coverage as an employee benefit. The cost of health insurance is a key factor driving the decisions of its purchasers; therefore, it often is employers who make the decisions about coverage and types of plans.

At the same time that the market is bringing pressure to hold down health care expenses, medical practices continue to face escalating costs. Employee salaries, rent, supplies, and equipment costs are all continuing to increase, whereas income remains relatively constant. In addition to these more or less normal increases in the cost of providing health care to patients, obstetrician–gynecologists in many markets are regularly facing double digit increases in liability insurance premiums, often to more than $100,000 per year.

During medical school and residency, physicians in the United States receive excellent training that enables them to provide superb medical care to patients, but the breadth and depth of the clinical knowledge and skill that must be acquired leave little time for developing the nonclinical aspects of practicing medicine. Although practice managers, accountants, and financial advisors gather and present relevant information, physicians need to know how to interpret and use that information. It is important for physicians to have the leadership and management skills needed to operate their practices like the businesses they are.

Recognizing this need, the Junior Fellow College Advisory Council recommended that the American College of Obstetricians and Gynecologists (ACOG) develop material for residents to help prepare them for the business and personal finance issues they will face after residency. In response to this recommendation, ACOG's Department of Health Economics developed this new publication titled *The Business of Medicine: An Essential Guide for Obstetrician–Gynecologists*. This publication covers a variety of topics, including getting started in practice, managing a practice, and personal finance issues. Although developed with the resident in mind, it also is useful for obstetrician–gynecologists already in practice who are looking for guidance on these topics.

In addition to *The Business of Medicine: An Essential Guide for Obstetrician–Gynecologists*, ACOG developed a companion guide to help with professional liability issues, *Professional Liability and Risk Management: An Essential Guide for Obstetrician–Gynecologists*, and a monograph to help obstetrician–gynecologists understand the principles of correct coding, *The Essential Guide to Coding in Obstetrics and Gynecology*. It is hoped that these three publications will complement one another and assist new physicians and others who seek additional understanding of these important nonclinical, but nevertheless essential, subjects and methods.

Albert L. Strunk, JD, MD, FACOG
Vice President, Fellowship Activities
The American College of Obstetricians and Gynecologists

THE BUSINESS OF MEDICINE

An Essential Guide for Obstetrician–Gynecologists

Chapter 1. **Planning for Practice**

Timetable for Making Decisions

There are a lot of decisions you must make as you plan to practice. A general idea of how much time you should allow for your move to a career in obstetric–gynecologic practice is shown in the following timetable for making decisions:

At 12 months ahead:

1. Start researching practice opportunities
2. Prepare your curriculum vitae and contact potential references
3. Narrow down your choices of practices
4. Begin gathering data on the communities and hospitals in your top choices

At 9 months ahead:

1. Make interview appointments
2. Go to interviews (take your significant other on the trip)
3. Choose advisors you need (eg, attorney, accountant, banker, real estate agent)
4. Make final decision and sign contract
5. Apply for state licensure; if already licensed in that state, inform licensing board of proposed address change
6. Apply for narcotic license from Drug Enforcement Administration
7. Apply for Medicare and Medicaid provider numbers
8. Apply for hospital medical staff privileges

You need to understand your own preferences before you can assess a location.

At 2–5 months ahead:

1. Look for housing
2. Apply for insurance coverage (liability, health, disability) if not provided by group

3. Arrange for child care, school enrollment in new location

At 2–4 weeks ahead:

1. Move to new location

TIP

In moving to a new location, give yourself 1 week longer than you think you will need.

Choosing a Location

You probably already have an idea of the part of the country where you would like to live and whether you prefer urban, rural, or suburban living. Before you begin zeroing in on specific practice opportunities, take time to talk with your family about the qualities that are important to you in a community.

Livability Factors: Physician Know Thyself

You need to understand your own preferences before you can assess a location. What aspects are just appealing, and what are deal-breakers? Is the number of sunny days per year more important than the presence of a top-rate symphony orchestra? Do you need a good school system or an airport with nonstop flights to Seattle?

Of the following community characteristics, which are most important to you?

- Job opportunities for your partner
- Proximity to family and friends
- Availability of affordable housing
- Housing availability close to your practice or hospital where you will take calls
- Traffic and commuting times
- Living costs
- Cultural and recreational offerings that match your interests
- Quality of schools
- Pollution, crime
- Proximity to a major airport

Medical Practice Factors

Choosing a place to practice adds another layer of community characteristics that are important. Check out the following attributes for any city you are considering for an obstetric–gynecologic practice:

- Population trends
- Patient demographics: age, income, diversity
- Number of births
- Patient-to-physician ratio
- Health of the economy—unemployment rates, growth industries
- Health insurance plans of largest employers

Options for Practice

Group Practice

There are pros and cons to joining a group practice (Box 1–1). If you join an obstetric–gynecologic group practice, usually you will start with an employment contract as a salaried employee. The agreement will specify the period and terms under which you will be offered a financial partnership (see Chapter 3 for more on contracts).

Group Structures

In addition to being either single-specialty or multispecialty, groups can have four different kinds of legal structures:

1. Professional Corporation. Forming a corporation can protect the physicians' personal assets from creditors. The physicians are shareholders and elect or appoint a board of directors made up of shareholders. In small groups, the physicians usually share responsibilities on the board; in larger groups they may elect officers with specific functions for running the corporation.

BOX 1–1 GROUP PRACTICE

Pros

- Immediate income; less risk
- Call duties are shared
- Greater fringe benefits
- Increased interaction and opportunity for consultation with colleagues
- More leverage with managed care plans (large groups)
- Less administrative burden for the individual and financial stability in changing market
- Economies of scale in service contracts, supplies
- Increased ability to purchase office space, include onsite diagnostic capabilities
- During vacation, the group continues to generate income

Cons

- Potential interpersonal conflict and competition
- Less independence and flexibility
- Lack of control of practice operations
- Pressure to refer patients to group physicians (multispecialty groups)
- Potential for clinic-type atmosphere in very large practice
- Governance may favor vested partners

2. Partnership. Two or more physicians are co-owners of the practice. Each partner carries liability for the actions of other partners. The physicians share expenses and divide up income under a predetermined formula.

3. Limited Liability Company. A limited liability company combines some of the characteristics of a corporation with some of the characteristics of a partnership.

4. Proprietorship. One physician is the owner, who employs other physicians.

A fifth arrangement is not truly a group practice, but a collection of solo practitioners who share office space, equipment, and staff. Each physician is an independent practice.

Large Versus Small

The larger the group, the more stability there is when the market is undergoing major changes. Large multispecialty practices may be able to offer more attractive benefit packages than single-specialty groups, but often pay lower salaries. The lower salaries usually reflect fewer working hours. Large groups also have the means to employ professional staff with the expertise and training to handle management tasks that fall to the physicians in a smaller group.

Typically, the larger the practice the more bureaucratic and policy driven it is. For the physician joining a group as an employee, a large group often has less flexibility in negotiating terms of the contract: they cannot make exceptions to the benefits offered, for example. In addition, the more physicians in the practice, the greater the potential for personality conflict.

Working Within a Group

Joining a group practice entails accepting the philosophy and an agreed-on work style of the group. Look for a group that matches what you want in a practice:

- Group size and diversity of members (age, sex, subspecialties)
- Group philosophy (toward finances, lifestyle, patient care)
- Perspectives on managed care, Medicare, Medicaid
- Patient mix (age, ethnic diversity)
- Number and types of procedures done
- Use (or planned use) of computers for appointments, billing, medical records, laboratory or prescription orders

Nonclinical Responsibilities

Although an individual physician in a group practice does not have the entire responsibility for practice management, as in a solo practice, the paperwork and administrative duties increase with the size of the practice. Some tasks may be assigned to physicians on a rotating basis, or, in large groups, a small workgroup or committee may handle them.

Expect to participate in one or more of the following nonclinical duties or oversight responsibilities:

- Peer review
- Marketing
- Teaching
- Administration (eg, coding oversight, staff supervision)
- Utilization review
- Managed care negotiations

Compensation

When you join a group, you usually are offered an employment contract with a guaranteed salary for the first year (or longer in some cases), which serves as a trial period for both parties. The road to partnership after the first year should be clear. Sometimes there is a buy-in requirement to become a full partner.

After the initial period of a guaranteed salary, income usually is based on a combination of salary plus a productivity formula used by the group. Although some groups distribute the net practice income equally among all partners, most calculate compensation based on productivity or the fees the physician generates from patients. Most group partners are compensated with a mixture of salary plus productivity.

Some compensation formulas take into account a number of factors in addition to productivity, such as seniority, call coverage, administrative responsibilities, teaching, and bringing in new patients. Each factor is assigned a different weight in the formula.

The income distributed among the partners is the net income—after expenses are deducted. How the group defines expenses is an important part of the compensation plan. In some groups, all the partners share the expenses evenly. In practices with more sophisticated accounting, fixed expenses, such as rent and utilities, are allocated to each physician according to usage, based on square footage, for example, or on full-time versus part-time work. Direct expenses—equipment or staff used exclusively by one physician—also may be allocated separately in large practices. Another way to allocate expenses is to charge expenses as a percentage of productivity: if the obstetrician–gynecologist generates 30% of the income, he or she is charged 30% of the expenses.

There are no right or wrong kinds of compensation formulas. It is important that you understand the compensation approach for any group you consider. See Chapters 4 and 7 for more details on contracts and negotiations.

Solo Practice

Starting a solo practice usually requires some personal and financial sacrifice at the beginning. Becoming established usually takes at least 3 years. The personal and financial rewards can be great, making solo practice a good choice for those who are risk-takers, have a long-term perspective, and value independence over security (Box 1–2).

You can set up a solo practice as a sole proprietorship or a professional corporation. Corporate status affords protection of your personal assets from debt or lawsuits, but setting it up and filing taxes are more complicated.

Location

Location—both the community and the specific office site—is an especially important factor to consider when starting a solo practice. Look for a community that can use another obstetrician–gynecologist. Research the demographics and medical resources of a location you are considering.

Starting a solo practice is more likely to be successful in a rural area because of the lack of competition. You also may have more control over your fees in a rural area because managed care organizations have more penetration in urban areas, and the solo physician has little negotiating strength there.

BOX 1–2 SOLO PRACTICE

Pros

- Independence and control
- No group politics
- Clinical autonomy
- Ability to change office hours and policies to meet patient needs
- Flexibility to tailor schedule to meet personal preferences and needs
- Pride of ownership

Cons

- Sole responsibility for start-up costs
- Less daily interaction and consultation with colleagues
- No economies of scale for service contracts, supplies
- Lack of leverage with managed care plans
- Must negotiate call duty with other practices
- Difficulty in obtaining coverage for vacation
- Sole responsibility for administrative tasks

In addition to researching the demographics and the medical resources, a practical tip is to call several obstetric–gynecologic practices for an appointment. If it takes 2–3 weeks to see a physician, there may be a market for another practice in town.

In choosing a practice site, look for a place close to the hospital where you will be affiliated and which will be convenient for patients. Make sure there is adequate parking. In a big city, be sure it is accessible by public transportation. If the area is expanding, consider whether new streets or changes in zoning could adversely affect your practice.

Finances

You will need to determine start-up costs, not only for furnishing an office but also for your first-year expenses. Plan to have at least the following information and documentation to approach a bank, a hospital, or other sources for loans:

- Your analysis of the market
- Cost of needed equipment, furniture, and office-space improvements
- Expense budget for 24 months, including staffing, rent, utilities, clinical and office supplies, insurance, professional conferences and dues, and advisors' fees
- Projected income for 24 months
- Your curriculum vitae and medical license

A formal business plan is the ideal mechanism to organize the information and gain credibility with potential lenders. Numerous publications are available on how to prepare a business plan, but your best bet is to retain an accountant or management consultant to help you.

What Is Involved With Starting Your Own Practice

You will need at least 12 months lead time to complete the many steps involved in starting a solo practice (Box 1–3). A comprehensive discussion of these tasks is beyond the scope of this book, but this overview will give you some idea of what is involved and the lead time you will need.

Buying a Practice

Purchasing an established practice rather than starting a solo practice from scratch offers an immediate source of income. Some experts estimate that buying an existing practice puts physicians 4–5 years ahead.

Consult a professional with experience in practice appraisals to help you determine the value of a practice you are considering buying. The sale price of a practice is determined by the value of the practice assets minus the practice liabilities:

- Assets include the building (if owned); equipment; furniture; supplies; and the value of the patient base, referred to as the "goodwill value." Goodwill value usually is

BOX 1–3 TIMETABLE FOR STARTING A SOLO PRACTICE*

One year before

1. Finalize decision about community in which you will practice
2. Choose your advisors: accountant, attorney, and management consultant
3. Develop a business plan
4. Identify sources of loans; contact potential lenders
5. Check on the deadline for being listed in the telephone book yellow pages

Nine months before

1. Research sites for office space and finalize your office location
2. Determine office layout and equipment and utility requirements
3. Shop for and obtain bids on office equipment and furnishings
4. Apply for loan or line of credit for start-up financing
5. Identify health insurance plans you want to participate in and apply for credentialing
6. Apply for employer identification number

Six months before

1. Research advertising modes and determine their deadlines
2. Finalize lease for office space and begin ordering furnishings

3. Begin to recruit office staff
4. Establish fees and set up your billing system
5. Determine your medical record system and order supplies needed
6. Determine your computer and technology needs and choose vendors
7. Set up an employee benefit package
8. Create your retirement plan

Three months before

1. Hire and train office staff
2. Order clinical and business supplies
3. Advertise opening of practice (eg, send announcements to pharmacies, notify local paper)
4. Set office policies, including a written manual
5. Establish office hours
6. Arrange for call coverage
7. Select insurance policies for you and your staff (professional liability, health, life, disability)

One month before

1. Move into office
2. Start accepting appointments

*These tasks are in addition to the general timeline for tasks to prepare for practice presented previously.

determined as a percentage of the previous year's gross income. It is important that this figure has been consistent or growing for the past 5 years and that it does not include monies from sources other than the practice.

- Liabilities are outstanding loans plus any taxes, salaries, and insurance premiums due.

Important considerations regarding the practice value include the sources of income (payer mix) and the ratio of net income to expenses. The key to a good valuation is getting a good estimate of the practice's future income.

Experts recommend that the buyer and seller work together for at least 6–9 months to ensure a smooth transition in transferring patient loyalty and maintaining consultative and hospital relationships.

Academic Practice

In an academic practice, the obstetric–gynecologic department does the recruiting, interviewing, and hiring of physicians on the obstetric–gynecologic service. At most institutions, you will be an employee on a salary with defined benefits and promotion opportunities.

Unless you have had significant practice experience, your first position in academic medicine will likely be as a clinical instructor, a junior faculty rank. The next steps in promotion are assistant professor, associate professor, and full professor.

Traditionally, tenure is granted to faculty at the associate professor level. However, institutions are moving away from including tenure in the academic career track. Some institutions have a limited number of tenured positions, and some are dropping tenured positions completely.

At some academic centers, physicians are part of a university physician group or private faculty practice plan. This entity represents the physicians in negotiating with the institution for physician salaries, professional liability insurance, and other benefits.

If you are interested in an academic career, talk with the faculty in your residency about the pros and cons of academic medicine (Box 1–4). Remember, however, that their experiences are not universal; policies, culture, and expectations vary widely among institutions and even among departments within a university.

Most academic appointments combine responsibilities for teaching, patient care, and clinical research. The trend in recent years has been to require more direct involvement in patient care. Different institutions may emphasize and reward different priorities, such as treating a large number of billable patients or bringing in grant money.

Following are some of the responsibilities of a faculty member:

- Patient care
- Classroom teaching
- Bedside training of medical students and residents
- Writing and research
- Committees and administration

Public Sector Positions

The public sector offers a variety of very different options for obstetrician–gynecologists, from research at the National Institutes of Health to general practice on an Indian reservation. Government employment, whether at the federal, state, or local level, often presents attractive employment packages for physicians that may include recruitment bonuses or student loan paybacks. The Federal Tort Claims Act offers some liability protection, an important benefit. In addition, the fringe benefits offered in government positions usually are excellent (Box 1–5).

U.S. Government

The U.S. Public Health Service offers a variety of opportunities to provide care to underserved women in both urban and rural settings. You can

---

BOX 1–4 ACADEMIC PRACTICE

Pros

- Part if not all of salary guaranteed
- Paid benefits, such as continuing medical education costs and travel, vacation, professional dues, sabbatical, journal subscriptions
- Diversity in responsibilities: patient care, teaching, writing, research
- Intellectually stimulating environment
- Interaction with and ready access to all specialties
- Challenging patient cases
- Opportunity to train the next generation of obstetrician–gynecologists
- Paid sabbatical after a period of years

Cons

- Lower salary than private practice
- Multiple chains of command and bureaucratic requirements that slow decisions or block innovation
- Competing demands for your energy and time in research, teaching, and clinical care
- Pressure to publish or pursue outside funding for research
- Political and turf battles
- Lack of autonomy and direct control over management decisions

BOX 1–5 PUBLIC-SECTOR POSITIONS

Pros

- Providing care regardless of patients' ability to pay
- Secure salary and benefits
- Defined retirement, leave time
- Less responsibility for running a practice and marketing
- Opportunity to serve women in real need (underserved areas and public hospitals)
- More defined and regular hours than in private practice
- Paid travel (in some positions)

Cons

- Lower income than in private practice
- Dealing with bureaucracy
- Lack of autonomy and control over practice policies
- Lack of choice in assigned locations (in some U.S. branches)

be either a civil service employee or part of the Commissioned Corps, a uniformed service of health professional officers headed by the U.S. Surgeon General.

These are two major services that are looking for obstetrician–gynecologists for underserved areas:

1. National Health Service Corps. When you commit to serve for 2 years, you are eligible to receive up to $50,000 to repay student loans. This is in addition to the salary and benefits that you negotiate directly with the community where you work.

2. Indian Health Service. The Indian Health Service places obstetrician–gynecologists in Indian and Alaskan Native communities throughout the United States. Committing to serve for 2 years at an approved site makes you eligible for a loan repayment program of up to $20,000 per year for health professional loans.

The U.S. government has many other agencies that hire physicians, including the U.S. military, the National Institutes of Health, the Federal Drug Administration, and the Centers for Disease Control and Prevention. Agencies that you may not associate with health care also need physicians. These are as wide-ranging as the Federal Bureau of Investigation and the Department of Education.

Other Public-Sector Positions

States, counties, and cities offer positions both in patient care and in administration. For administrative or policy positions, additional education will be helpful, and you should consider pursuing degrees in public health, hospital administration, public policy, environmental policy, or public administration.

If you are interested in public service or a career in health policy or administration, check with the following organizations for available opportunities:

- Public hospitals: Clinics in large urban public hospitals as well as smaller community hospitals funded by cities and counties
- State and county health departments
- World Health Organization

Locum Tenens

Working as a locum tenens means you fill in for another obstetrician–gynecologist temporarily, usually to cover for vacation or illness or while a practice is recruiting a replacement for someone who left. (The term *locum tenens* is Latin for "one who holds the place.") Length of assignments can vary from a few weeks to many months.

Practicing in temporary assignments can be a good way to investigate types of practices—urban, rural, large group, and small group (Box 1–6). It also is a way to work part time. For example, you may choose to work locum tenens for 6 months of the year and travel the rest of the time.

Finding locum tenens assignments is done through national placement firms. Hospitals and practices that need an obstetrician–gynecologist to fill in pay the locum tenens agency a fee to find a well-qualified obstetrician–gynecologist to work for a designated period. The following are two types of locum tenens placement firms:

1. Clearinghouse agency. Practices needing coverage contact the firm, which sends them your curriculum vitae. The agency serves as the intermediary and the employer interviews you and contracts with you directly. The locum tenens agency usually arranges for your travel and housing. In this arrangement, you are an independent contractor, so taxes are not withheld from your paycheck, and you have the responsibility to pay your federal and state taxes and Social Security. Because you are a contractor and not an employee, there are no fringe benefits, such as health and liability insurance or a retirement plan.

2. Full-service agency. You are an employee of the locum tenens company, which withholds taxes; pays the employer portion of Social Security; and provides benefits, such as professional liability insurance.

A contract with a locum tenens agency should clearly address payment terms, coverage of expenses, lodging, and professional liability insur-ance. It is especially important to know what kind of liability insurance coverage is provided. See Chapter 6 for details about the difference between occurrence insurance and claims-made insurance.

The locum tenens agency is retained by the practice. Thus, their goal is to meet the practice's needs, not yours. Physicians experienced in locum tenens assignments advise not to make a long-term commitment to an assignment at first because the situation may not be agreeable. To keep from being locked in, try to have an assignment limited to 1 or 2 weeks initially, with an option to extend it.

The agreement with the locum tenens company should specify minimal standards for the type of lodging you expect. You may want to specify a small apartment with access to a kitchen. Typically, your food expenses are not covered, so this can spare you from eating out all the time.

Hospital Sponsorship

A hospital may buy practices or offer financial help to physicians through a variety of arrangements. The hospital may be in an underserved area that needs obstetrician–gynecologists or in a competitive environment where it is trying to guarantee referrals for inpatient services. There are pros and cons to working under hospital sponsorship (Box 1–7).

Independent Contractor

In one type of arrangement, you have your own practice as an independent contractor, and the hospital provides financial assistance. Following are some of the kinds of financial benefits that may be offered:

- Recruitment and practice assistance. The hospital may pay for your house-hunting and relocation costs and pay for your practice expenses for a period, such as 6 months.

- Income guarantee. The hospital will guarantee you a certain income to help you get started. Usually the agreement is for 1 year.

BOX 1–6 LOCUM TENENS POSITIONS

Pros

- Potential to work less than full time and have extended time off
- Opportunity to check out different geographic locations and types of practices
- Opportunity to have income while looking for a full-time practice
- High rate of pay

Cons

- Lack of sense of permanency, of having your own practice or patient base
- No ability to check out a practice before you arrive for the assignment

For example, the hospital may guarantee an income of $150,000; if you earn $100,000 from practice revenue, the hospital will pay you the difference. The stipulations for you to pay the hospital back may take different forms: agreeing to stay in the area for a specified period, paying back the money (sometimes without interest), or providing services to the hospital.

- Office and equipment. The hospital may offer you a lease agreement for office space or purchase equipment and lease it back to you at a favorable rate. Another option is for the hospital to advance you the money to purchase equipment at a favorable interest rate.

- Practice services. The hospital may offer services such as recruiting office staff or providing billing and accounting services.

Financial assistance that you receive from the hospital that does not have to be paid back is treated as taxable income by the Internal Revenue Service.

Employee

In a second type of hospital relationship, the hospital owns the obstetric–gynecologic practice and pays the physicians a salary to practice. Typically, the hospital runs the practice—hiring the office staff and handling billing arrangements with third-party payers. As owner of the practice (and payer of the bills), the hospital requires its

approval of the selection and purchase of equipment you wish to use in practice.

Practice arrangements available with hospitals are constantly changing as market forces change. Many hospitals now offer a compensation package that combines salary plus productivity incentives, such as income generated, patent satisfaction surveys, or cost-effective resource utilization.

Management and Administration

Many opportunities exist outside clinical practice. Your medical training and perspective are valuable to corporations, nonprofit organizations, and government agencies such as:

- Institute of Medicine and other government agencies

- Pharmaceutical companies

- Environmental organizations

- Managed care and insurance companies

- Health care foundations and medical associations

- Think tanks

- Risk management companies

If you are interested in a nonclinical career, either now or in the future, many resources are available to help you assess your personality and skill compatibility and to provide more information about opportunities and how to prepare for them.

If you wish to practice clinically first, volunteer to serve on hospital committees, speak to community organizations, and participate in the administrative tasks of your practice. Hone your interpersonal skills and public speaking, learn how to be effective in planning and running meetings, and become a student of small-group dynamics. All these areas of experience will serve you well in the nonclinical arena. Chapter 7 covers aspects of leadership, communication, and team building.

The American College of Obstetricians and Gynecologists provides several programs that teach leadership and management skills. One is the postgraduate course "Advanced Quality

Improvement and Management Skills for Leaders in Women's Health Care," which includes sessions on finance and accounting, changing behavior, management skills, and assessing return on investment.

The American College of Obstetricians and Gynecologists also offers an annual conference, Future Leaders in Obstetrics and Gynecology, designed especially for Junior Fellows. Topics include media relations, meeting effectiveness, interpersonal skills, team development, and project management.

The American College of Physician Executives is probably the best-known single organization focusing on management careers specifically for physicians. It offers education, consultation, and publications for physicians looking for nonclinical careers.

Part-Time Positions

Look for an employer that makes your part-time contribution worthwhile. Working part time is possible in virtually any of the practice types described previously, but jobs can be structured in myriad ways. Identify your own goals first and then find a part-time arrangement that meets your goals or approach a practice and present your ideas.

Before you begin, obtain explicit information about how many patients you are expected to see during your hours. More important, find out what nonclinical duties are expected—record-keeping and data entry requirements, as well as attendance at group or hospital meetings and participation in quality improvement or group education activities.

TIP

It usually is better to work 2 or 3 full days rather than 4 or 5 half days. Half days have a way of expanding into extra hours.

Compensation

Income arrangements for part-time work may be based on daily or hourly rates or a percentage of income generated or some formula to measure productivity. When negotiating for a part-time position, find out how what you are offered compares to what full-time physicians receive. Most practices have compensation policies that favor full-time physicians because they are more valuable to a group. Because overhead expenses are approximately the same for part-time and full-time physicians, there is not a linear relationship between hours worked and income after expenses.

If your compensation is based on productivity, you can control your earnings. However, if you are on a salary, you may have to negotiate.

Negotiating the Terms

These topics can serve as negotiating areas to reach a win-win agreement for part-time work:

- Salary. Do the math; find out if part-time pay is commensurate with full-time pay (50% hours = 50% pay).

- Liability insurance. Some carriers prorate premiums or offer a discount for part-time physicians; this may be based on the number of deliveries, hours worked, or some other formula; if the group's insurance company will not offer a lower rate for part-time work, you can buy your own insurance and use this for negotiating leverage. In addition, your own policy may be more transferable if you change jobs.

- Practice expenses. For a practice with both full- and part-time physicians, allocated practice expenses should be divided between fixed expenses (eg, rent, utilities, furniture) and variable expenses (eg, supplies, office staff). Point out that it is inequitable to the part-time physician to share equal expenses with the full-time physicians.

- Fringe benefits. Vacation, continuing medical education allowances, and insurance coverage might be prorated or not offered at all to part-timers. Leave time for continuing education and vacation are part of the mix of benefits and compensation that you can negotiate. It is arguable that you should receive full continuing medical education benefits because of the importance (and requirements) for continuing education.

- Partnership opportunity. Part-time physicians often are not given an ownership position. If you seek this, especially if you think you will move to full-time status later, try for an agreement that will give you credit for the time spent working part time.

Shared Practice

Two physicians can divide a full-time position, working alternate days, dividing the schedule, or splitting the patient load in a way that suits them. Your practice styles and philosophy must be compatible for a shared schedule to work: an obstetrician–gynecologist who typically spends 20 minutes with a patient for an office visit will be poorly matched with an obstetrician–gynecologist who would take 5 minutes for the same patient.

Beware the Expanding Hours

Many physicians have found that their dream of working 20 or 30 hours per week is just that—a dream. Physicians, especially, are subject to the "expanding work" phenomenon, for several reasons:

- Physicians are self-selected overachievers.

- Providing medical care does not lend itself to tidy boundaries; you cannot always walk away when the clock says "time's up."

- Health care delivery is increasingly complex: insurance, managed care, and hospital requirements are among the demands on your time in addition to patient care.

Talk to as many physicians as you can who have done what you are trying to do—whether part-time patient care, back-up coverage for a group, or a part-time administrative or research position. Make a list of the challenges they mention. As much as possible, address these with your employer when you begin the job.

Sources of Information

Location

- Sperling's Best Places—Gives school statistics, crime rates, climate profiles, and cost-of-living data: www.bestplaces.net

- *Places Rated Almanac:* Ranks metropolitan areas in the United States and Canada on cost of living, transportation, education, health care, climate, and more. It has a quiz that helps you identify what factors are most important to you in a place to live.

- Crime statistics: The Federal Bureau of Investigation's *Uniform Crime Reports* are available online at www.fbi.gov/ucr/ucr.htm

- Regional planning commissions

- Census reports: quickfacts.census.gov

- State departments of tourism and business development

- State and city Chambers of Commerce: Every state has a chamber of commerce; community chambers often have a newcomer's packet that includes maps, business statistics, and other information about the city and state

- Local and state medical societies

- Real estate companies in the area

- Obstetrician–gynecologists in the area

- Hospital marketing or planning department; American Hospital Directory has a free online directory with links to hospital web sites at www.ahd.com.

Group Practice

- Medical Group Management Association: www.mgma.com

- American Medical Association: www.ama-assn.org

Solo Practice

- "Practice Valuation: A Primer for Obstetrician–Gynecologists," published by the American College of Obstetricians and Gynecologists: www.acog.org

- American Society of Appraisers, Business Valuation Division: www.bvappraiers.org

- American Academy of Family Physicians: www.aafp.org

- *Starting a Medical Practice: The Physician's Handbook for Successful Practice Start-Up*, published by the American Medical Association: www.ama-assn.org

- *Medical Economics* series of seven articles, "Starting a Practice," March–July 2004: www.memag.com

- National Association of Healthcare Consultants: www.healthcon.org

- *Starting a Medical Practice from the Ground Up*, published by the American Academy of Family Physicians: www.aafp.org/catalog or 800-944-0000

Academic Practice

- *Academic Medicine*—Monthly journal of the Association of American Medical Colleges: www.aamc.org

- Association of Professors in Gynecology and Obstetrics: www.apgo.org

- Council of Residency Educators in Ob-Gyn: www.acog.org

Public Sector Positions

- Indian Health Service: www.ihs.gov

- National Health Service Corps: nhsc.bhpr.hrsa/gov

- National Association of Public Hospitals and Health Systems: www.naph.org

- California Association of Public Hospitals and Health Systems: www.caph.org

- American Public Health Association: www.apha.org

- Association of Schools of Public Health: www.asph.org

- National Association for Public Health Statistics and Information Systems: www.naphsis.org

- World Health Organization: www.who.int/en

Locum Tenens

- National Association of Locum Tenens Organizations: www.nalto.org

Hospital Sponsorship

- American College of Physician Career Resource Center: www.acponline.org/careers

- American Hospital Directory: www.ahd.com

- Medical Group Management Association: www.mgma.org

Management and Administration

- The American College of Obstetricians and Gynecologists: www.acog.org

- American College of Physician Executives: www.acpe.org

- *Leaving the Bedside: The Search for a Nonclinical Medical Career*, published by the American Medical Association: www.ama-assn.org

- *Planning for a Successful Career Transition*, published by the American Medical Association: www.ama-assn.org

Part-Time Positions

- American Medical Association: www.ama-assn.org

- How and When to Find a Job Share Partner: www.momMD.com (web site focused exclusively on women in medicine and their issues)

- "Part-Time Practice: Making It Work": www.aafp.org

Chapter 2. Finding a Position

Resources for Finding a Position

Networking

The more people you tell that you are looking for a position, the better your chance of finding a connection to someone who knows someone with an opening. Be as specific as you can about your goal. Have a concise description that you can easily convey, such as "a five- or six-person practice in a medium-sized city in New England" or "a part-time position anywhere in Colorado."

You should start with your residency director and attending physicians, along with past graduates of your program. If you already live in the area where you want to practice, include individuals who work in health care in your network. Talk to pharmacists, hospital employees, medical equipment sales representatives, and pharmaceutical representatives about opportunities. Give them a business card or write down your contact information so they can reach you later. The American College of Obstetricians and Gynecologists' district meetings, held every fall, and the national Annual Clinical Meeting held in April or May are great places to network.

Medical Journals

Medical journals can be good resources for finding positions:

- *Obstetrics & Gynecology* (the Green Journal) and other obstetric–gynecologic journals publish classified advertisements for physician positions.

- *JAMA* and the *New England Journal of Medicine* list positions available.

- *Academic Medicine*, published by the Association of American Medical Colleges, has classified advertisements for open academic positions.

The easiest way to find out about a medical society's services and contact information is to go to the medical society web site.

Internet Job Banks

Many companies, physician journals, medical societies, and hospitals have set up physician job databases that are free to the physician looking for a position (the practice seeking a physician pays a fee to list the position). Some job banks focus on positions in one state or region whereas others list positions nationwide. Virtually all job banks are now online and have a mechanism for you to register, send your curriculum vitae directly to a recruiting practice, and receive e-mail notices of new openings.

TIP

Have business cards printed with your contact information to be sure someone can easily get in touch with you.

Hospitals

Large hospitals often have information about practice opportunities in the areas they serve. You can call the hospital and ask for the medical staff office or the staff that handles physician recruitment.

State Medical Societies

Many state medical societies and a few large county medical societies offer placement services. They may have an online job bank, run classified advertisements in their medical journal or newspaper or both. The easiest way to find out about a medical society's services and contact information is to go to the medical society web site.

Physician Recruiters and Placement Services

There are hundreds of physician recruiting firms that can help you find a position. Some recruiting firms limit their work to a certain state or region. Some hospitals or large organizations have staff recruiters.

A recruiter talks to you about your preferences and presents you with opportunities that match your goals (Box 2–1). If you want to pursue an opening, the recruiter will help you set up an interview and give you advice about how best to present yourself. Most important, the recruiter will give you helpful feedback after the interview.

You do not pay a fee to a recruiter. A professional recruiter is paid by the practice or hospital that is recruiting a physician. Professional standards for recruiting that address confidentiality,

BOX 2–1   RECRUITMENT FIRMS

Pros

- Does the leg work of searching for you
- May have positions not advertised elsewhere
- May offer bonus for placement
- Provides helpful information about the practice and community
- Will give advice on interview preparation and may arrange your travel
- Will provide feedback about your interview

Cons

- Caution: There is a negative reaction against recruitment firms in some of the most desirable markets*
- Caution: The most desirable positions are not likely to be listed with recruitment firms*
- Caution: Some practices refuse to receive resumes submitted by recruitment firms*
- Not comprehensive—many practices will not list with recruitment firms because of high fees
- May oversell a position or gloss over some negatives
- May require you to stay in a position for several years

*Note: These cautions apply particularly to private, fee-for-service recruiting firms; they are not directed toward staff recruiters employed by hospitals or large health care organizations.

fees, and conflicts of interest are available from the National Association of Physician Recruiters.

Practices who use a recruitment firm or placement service sometimes pay a flat retainer fee, but the fee often is contingent on filling the position. Contingency fees may be equal to 20–25% of the first-year income of the position. The recruiter is working for the practice that is paying the fee and may hold back or minimize negative information about the community or the practice.

Listed as follows are good questions to ask a recruiter:

- How long has your firm been in this business?
- What is your experience with obstetrician–gynecologists?

- How many obstetrician–gynecologists have you placed in the past year?

- Are you being paid on a contingency basis?

- Have you visited the practice in question?

It is okay to work with more than one recruiter. You should be honest with all of them about all the ways you are trying to find a position. When you find a position, you should promptly notify all the recruiters who have worked with you.

Sometimes a recruiter will offer a bonus to you if you take a position. These offers are most often made for positions in underserved areas that have hard-to-fill physician openings. Typically, such a bonus has some conditions, such as a commitment to stay in the position for several years. If you do not stay, you have to pay back the bonus or a portion of it or pay for recruiting your replacement.

TIP

A good recruiter will have personally visited the practice represented.

Curriculum Vitae Preparation

Prospective employers and partners usually will see your curriculum vitae before they meet you, so it needs to do the best possible job of presenting you effectively. A resume is the term used for a short curriculum vitae; the difference between the two is primarily semantic because both serve the same purpose—to summarize your relevant education and experience.

If you are just graduating from residency, your curriculum vitae will be brief, one or two pages at the most. Do not add fluff or be verbose just to make it longer. The goal in preparing your curriculum vitae is to give an easy-to-follow summary of who you are, presenting your strengths and qualifications in the most positive light. Tips for writing your curriculum vitae are shown in Box 2–2.

Some aspects of your curriculum vitae depend on your personal preference—whether to include hobbies or personal interests, for example, and whether to use abbreviations (B.S. or Bachelor of

Science). Some advisors say not to include personal interests but others suggest it creates a more well-rounded picture. These variables are up to you; you may even want to make changes in your curriculum vitae for different recipients.

Most consultants advise not to include date of birth, marital status, ethnicity, race, or religion on your curriculum vitae. Recruiters point out that the inclusion of these data could make a potential employer vulnerable to charges of discrimination if they screen you out of the interview process.

In listing your education and work experience, make sure any gaps in time are accounted for. If you had a break—whether it was traveling, working as a waitress, parenting, or trying to write a book—include it, with dates. List it in the appropriate section (Employment or Personal Information, for example).

You should have print copies of your curriculum vitae to mail and take to interviews, but you will want an electronic version to revise, e-mail, and copy and paste in online job banks. If you have your curriculum vitae prepared professionally, be sure you are given an electronic version.

Fax and e-mail your curriculum vitae to a friend or to yourself to be sure it is readable when received. If asked to e-mail your curriculum vitae to a prospective employer, confirm that the recipient can open the attachment (such as a Word or a PDF document).

TIP

In describing responsibilities or projects, use action verbs that convey leadership and management skills, such as established, managed, formed, conducted, led, presented, assessed, improved, revised, planned, oversaw, directed, and developed.

Cover Letter

Always include a cover letter when sending your curriculum vitae. Do not use a form letter—research the practice opportunity and tailor your letter according to the job. Your cover letter should be brief (no more than one page, usually

BOX 2–2 WRITING YOUR CURRICULUM VITAE

Format

- Use a font that is simple and conservative. The font size should be at least 12 (smaller than that does not fax well).
- Be generous with margins and white space.
- Make the headings boldface and larger than the text.
- Use bullet points for lists.
- Be consistent in use of abbreviations and capitalization (eg, use the same format for inclusive years: 2001–2004 or 2001–04).
- Proofread it carefully and ask another individual to do so; it must be letter-perfect.
- Print it or photocopy it on good-quality white or light-colored paper (cream or ivory, not a pastel color).
- Buy envelopes that match the paper for use when mailing it.

Name and address

- Use one address, home or business
- Include e-mail address
- List all telephone numbers at which you can take calls during regular business hours or that have an answering machine: home, cell, pager, and fax

Education and training

- List institution(s), degree(s), and date(s) of degree(s) or years attended
- State your undergraduate major
- Do not include high school

Employment experience

- Start with most recent first and work backwards
- Include job title, employer, city and state, dates (month and year) of employment
- Use active verbs to briefly describe your responsibilities or accomplishments
- Include volunteer work if it was relevant; state that it was volunteer or pro bono

Licensure and certification

- List the states where you are licensed to practice medicine (do not include license numbers)
- List Drug Enforcement Administation date of licensure (do not include license number)
- List board certification(s) or where you are in the process of seeking certification

Military service

- State branch, years of service, and rank at discharge
- List locations where stationed

Professional society memberships

- Include national and local memberships
- List offices or leadership positions held

Awards and honors

- Section can be omitted and individual awards listed with education or work experience
- List professional or academic awards and scholarships
- Do not go back further than college
- If the award is not nationally known, include a brief description

Special skills

- Include personal skills that could be important in practice, such as fluency in other languages or advanced computer skills

Extracurricular activities (optional)

- List areas of interest, such as hobbies or nonmedical organizations, in which you participate
- List specific projects if relevant

Publications and presentations

- Include presentations and dates
- Use bibliography format for publications of which you are author or co-author
- Include works in progress

References

- Omit names and state "Personal and professional references supplied on request."
- When you do provide names and contact information for references, let your references know who might be contacting them.

three paragraphs) and include the following information:

- Date

- Name and address of prospective employer

- Salutation. Always identify an individual; never use a generic "Dear Doctor" or "Dear Sir"

- Opening paragraph. State what position you are seeking and a description of how you heard about it. If you met this individual before, mention it here ("I enjoyed talking with you about your practice at the District IV dinner in Ashgrove").

- Second paragraph. Highlight the expertise and special interests you would bring to this position. You do not need to repeat what is in your curriculum vitae, but expand on it. Focus on accomplishments or interests you think would be valuable to this practice.

- Closing paragraph. Thank the employer for taking the time to consider you. Ask for an opportunity for an interview. If you know little about the practice, ask for practice details or brochures.

- Signature. Sign your name legibly, in blue or black ink.

- Your contact information. Below your signature, repeat your full name, address, and contact information, as shown on your curriculum vitae.

Interview Process

If you have two or three practices that you are seriously considering, decide which one you think is your best option and schedule that interview last. You can then use the other practices as a base for comparison, and you will have the chance to practice your interviewing skills. Because you will already know what the other practices have to offer, you also will be able to ask focused questions in preparation for contract negotiations.

TIP

Make copies of your licenses and registrations and designate one place to keep everything together. You will need them—time and again—for credentialing and interviewing.

Do Your Homework

Before the interview, check the web sites and, if possible, brochures or other literature produced by the practice, the community, and the hospital(s). Try to find out how long the practice has been recruiting for this position and how soon they would like a new physician to begin work.

Make a list of topics you want to discuss and refer to it during the interview. Your preparation will impress the interviewers and serve as a tool for exchanging information during the interview.

Telephone Interview

A telephone interview is a likely first step before the practice commits to setting up a lengthy interview, especially if it involves travel expenses. If you are contacted for more information, avoid the pitfall of starting to answer a lot of questions when you are not prepared. Set up an appointment to talk when you can focus your full attention.

A telephone interview is an opportunity for each party to screen the other and find out answers to basic questions. It is not the time for detailed negotiation. Never consider an offer without visiting the practice.

In-Person Interview

The interview process may cover 2 or even 3 days and should include a tour of the hospital(s). If the interview process is scheduled for 1 day, take a second day on your own to look at the community.

The prospective employer usually pays your travel and hotel expenses. Your significant other should go with you to look at the community, potential jobs and housing, and participate in any social functions planned with the group. If you have children, leave them at home. You can ask if expenses also will be paid for your spouse or partner.

TIPS

- Be on time. If you are driving to an unfamiliar area, make a trial run to be sure you know the way and where to park.
- Act naturally. Although interviews can be stressful, remember that it is in your best interest to convey an honest version of yourself. Do not pretend to be someone you are not.
- Do not rush. Remember that it is okay to pause and think before answering a question.
- Use complete sentences. A simple "yes" or "no" answer to questions will not tell them much; they want to get to know you.

Plan Ahead

Ask for an agenda before the interview. Unless it is a very large group, you should meet all of the partners and office staff. You also should determine who is in charge of negotiations.

Appropriate interview dress for women is a suit or business dress. Men should wear a suit or sports jacket and tie. If a social function is planned, ask what dress would be appropriate; do not assume that a dinner will be formal—it could be an outdoor barbecue.

Ask what kinds of references are requested and take your list of references with contact information. Alert your references that someone may be contacting them.

Take extra copies of your curriculum vitae, statistics of procedures you have done, and your list of topics to discuss. Use an attractive folder with a note pad to hold your paperwork and to use for taking notes during the interview.

On-site Investigation

During your visit, you will be asked a lot of questions. Some typical questions are shown in Box 2–3. In addition, you should confirm information you have researched and ask additional questions. To reach your goal of having a clear picture of the practice when you leave, listen closely to what you are told and ask follow-up

BOX 2–3 QUESTIONS TO EXPECT

Take time to think about how you would answer some typical questions:

- What were the emphasis and philosophy of your training program?
- Why did you choose your training program, and what other programs did you consider?
- What did you like best and least about your training?
- Describe your ideal practice situation.
- How could you add to our practice?
- Describe your clinical experience.
- What are your goals 5 and 10 years from now?
- Why did you choose obstetrics and gynecology as a specialty?
- What are your strengths and weaknesses?
- How would your colleagues/nurses describe your character and practice style?
- How would you describe yourself, both personally and professionally?
- Describe a mistake you made with a patient.
- When do you want to start practice?
- What kind of salary are you looking for?
- What do you like to do in your free time?
- What experience have you had with managed care plans?
- Why do you want to live here?

questions (Box 2–4). At the beginning or on the first day of interviews, focus your questions on the practice and community—the physicians, patients, and office administration. On the second day or in the closing interview, you can address topics of practice finances, productivity expectations, and compensation.

In addition to asking a lot of questions, you should ask to see any managed care reports, including physician profiles or other audits. Note the practice's medical record system and ask for permission to review a few patient records (randomly chosen).

BOX 2-4 QUESTIONS TO ASK

Physicians and patients

- What is the total patient volume and mix of patients—ages, languages spoken?
- What are the practice statistics for deliveries and types of surgery?
- Does the group provide coverage for nurse midwives and family physicians?
- How is call coverage handled?
- How are new patients assigned?
- How long has each physician been with the group? Have any physicians left the group in the past 5 years? Why did they leave?
- What are the profiles of the group members—training, certification, years in practice?
- How is the quality of care evaluated?
- What are the philosophies of the group or individual members regarding elective abortions?
- What activities—with the community, the American College of Obstetricians and Gynecologists, or medical society—do group members participate in?
- What has been the group's experience in medical liability claims? Are any suits pending?

Medical and hospital resources

- What consultation is available?
- What are the strengths and weaknesses of the hospital(s) used?
- How is the hospital obstetric–gynecologic department structured, and how does it function?
- What level is the hospital nursery?
- How are operating rooms and procedure rooms scheduled?

The community

- What do you like best about living here?
- How is the traffic around the office and hospital?

Business and finances

- What is the legal structure of the group?
- Is the office owned or leased?
- What is the group's market area—geographically and in population?
- How many obstetric–gynecologic practices are in the community?

- What is the group's share of the obstetric–gynecologic market?
- What is the overall payer mix?
- Do all the group physicians participate in Medicare?
- How is billing handled?
- What percentage of accounts receivable are collected and what is the lag time?
- What managed care contracts are in place and are others being negotiated?
- Are the managed care panels open to me?
- What are the total income and overhead expenses of the group?
- How is income divided among the partners?
- Is a data collection system in place for procedures or other aspects of the practice?
- How long do patients usually have to wait for an office appointment?
- Does the practice have (or have plans for) computerized appointment scheduling, medical records, patient e-mail access, or laboratory and prescription orders?
- How is patient satisfaction measured?
- Does the practice have a standard policy about extending professional courtesy?
- How have you determined you need another physician?
- What changes are under way or contemplated that would affect the practice (eg, medical staff or hospital changes, moving the office, adding subspecialists to the group)

Compensation package

- What is the compensation offered, and how will it be paid?
- How is productivity defined and calculated?
- Will I be eligible for any productivity bonus during the first year?
- What are the nonclinical responsibilities?
- What input will I have in decision making for the practice, including office staffing and policies, clinical issues, and business decisions?
- What type of medical liability insurance is offered?
- Will the practice pay for the medical liability insurance?
- Will the practice pay for the medical liability tail policy?
- What fringe benefits are provided?
- What is the route to partnership and how is partnership defined?

Closely observe the office staff while you are there. Notice how they interact with you, the other physicians, the patients, and each other. Note how the telephone is answered and how patients are greeted, registered, and checked out. Ask to see the office policy manual.

You also should gain a clear picture of the financial health of the practice. You may feel awkward asking probing questions about the practice's financial condition, but most practices will welcome your questions. The timing of such questions is important; do not delve into this topic unless you are serious about pursuing an employment relationship and the practice has expressed a serious interest in you.

Plan to leave the interview with a clear understanding of your expected caseload, call schedule, nonclinical duties, and compensation, as well as a profile of the patient mix and care provided. You should determine if your practice philosophy, personal values, and work style are compatible with those of the other physicians in the practice. Finally, find out if there will be follow-up interviews and when an offer will be made.

Follow-up Letter

After the interview, send a brief thank-you letter that includes the following components:

- A thank-you for the opportunity to learn about the practice

- Specific mention of one or more aspects of the practice or community that impressed you

- List of expenses, unless you have been given a standard form to complete; attach copies of receipts

- Indication of the next steps (eg, you have more interviews scheduled, you are looking forward to their decision, or you will provide additional information they requested)

Assessing a Position

It is a good idea to put in writing an assessment of each practice you consider. Within a day or

two of your interview, use your notes to summarize your impressions and key points about the practice and the community. You may want to create a list of specific factors and your personal rating of each practice you visit (Box 2–5). In addition, you should be aware of potential problems. Warning signs of possible problems include:

- Refusal to show you financial data

- A pattern of frequent physician or staff turnover in the past 2 years

- No goals in place for the practice

- Widely disparate practice styles within the group

When seriously considering taking a position, retain professional advisors to help you analyze the practice's financial condition and the terms of an offer. The role of advisors is addressed further in Chapter 3.

TIP

The culture of a practice—the attitudes, interpersonal dynamics, and efficiency of the office—is a critical element of job satisfaction that will not be written into a contract.

Sources of Information

Resources for Finding a Position

- The American College of Obstetricians and Gynecologists; Career Connection: www.acog.org

- American Hospital Directory: www.ahd.com

- National Association of Physician Recruiters: www.napr.org or 800-726-5613

- *New England Journal of Medicine*: nejmjobs.org

- PracticeLink Physician & Healthcare Job Bank: www.practicelink.com

BOX 2–5 CHECKLIST FOR ASSESSING A POSITION

Practice characteristics
- Demographics of patient base
- Clinical profile of patients
- Clinical and surgical skills of the physicians
- Procedures and deliveries
- Consultation patterns
- Relations with hospital administration
- Experience with liability claims

Compatibility with group
- Size of group and profiles of individuals (age, sex, specialty)
- Priorities and values regarding lifestyle, income
- Attitudes toward vaginal birth after cesarean delivery, operative deliveries, consultation, elective abortion
- Involvement with community
- Involvement with medical societies and the American College of Obstetricians and Gynecologists
- Expectations about socializing with group members

Office facility and procedures
- Overall appearance
- Office hours and patient scheduling
- Layout and spaciousness of examination rooms and offices
- Medical equipment
- Patient flow
- Medical record system
- Arrangements for ancillary services
- Computer equipment, software, and support
- Written policies
- Distance to hospitals

Office staffing
- Number, roles, and qualifications
- Turnover
- Efficiency
- Role in patient education

Business specifics
- Legal structure and governance of group
- Size of market area (geographic and population)
- Obstetric–gynecologic competition in market area
- Fee schedule

- Payer mix of patients
- Participation in Medicare
- Contracts with managed care plans and integrated systems
- Billing and collection systems
- Total income and expenses
- Percentage of gross charges collected
- Aging of receivables, especially percentage older than 90 days
- Division of expenses and income among partners

Hospital characteristics
- Financial stability
- Plans for change, particularly related to obstetrics and gynecology
- Size and level
- Surgical suites
- Emergency services
- Anesthesiology services
- Laboratory services
- Fetal imaging services
- Genetic counseling
- Labor and delivery unit
- Nursery facilities and neonatal consultation
- Lactation consultant
- Nursing: nurse-to-patient ratios, morale, use of floaters and agency nurses

Compensation package
- Clinical responsibilities
- Administrative responsibilities
- Productivity expectation
- Call-duty requirements
- Salary
- Relocation allowance
- Buy-in agreement and specifics about partnership opportunity
- Continuing medical education: paid leave time, expense allowance
- Vacation time
- Retirement plan
- Health insurance
- Life insurance
- Medical liability insurance coverage
- Incentives or bonuses

- Physiciannet: www.physiciannet.com
- Physician Employment: www.physemp.com
- American Medical Group Association: www.amga.org
- *Academic Physician & Scientist:* www.acphysci.com
- CareerMD: www.careermd.com
- National Health Service Corps: nhsc.bhpr.hrsa/gov
- Indian Health Service: www.ihs.gov
- *Obstetrics & Gynecology* (the Green Journal) and other obstetric–gynecologic journals
- *Academic Medicine,* published by the Association of American Medical Colleges

Curriculum Vitae and Cover Letter Preparation

- *The Physician's Resume and Cover Letter Workbook: Tips and Techniques for a Dynamic Career Presentation,* by Sharon L. Yenney: www.amapress.com or 800-621-8335

Interview Process

- *The Physician in Transition: Managing the Job Interview,* by Donald L. Double: www.amapress.com or 800-621-8335

Assessing a Position

- *Physician Compensation and Production Survey,* published annually by the Medical Group Management Association (reports survey results for both academic and private practice; it costs several hundred dollars, so check your medical or hospital library): www.mgma.com or 877-275-6462
- *Practice Patterns of Obstetrics/Gynecology, 2003,* published by the American Medical Association (reports data from 2001–02 survey on obstetric–gynecologic revenue, expenses, weeks worked, and hospital utilization): www.amapress.com or 800-621-8335
- *Profile of Ob-Gyn Practice,* published by the American College of Obstetricians and Gynecologists (reports 2003 survey data on obstetric–gynecologic average hours worked, procedures, and patient visits): www.acog.org or 800-673-8444 (ask for the Practice Management Department)

Chapter 3.   Selecting and Using Professional Advisors

They Are Worth It

Professional advice can help you in numerous aspects of medical practice. You may be tempted to rely on your own research and informal advice from colleagues and family about financial and legal transactions, but experienced physicians attest to the value of seeking professional consultation from the outset. Professionals cost money, but they pay off in the long run; getting out of a bad contract or redoing your financial plans after faulty structures have been established can be costly.

If you are starting your own practice, the three key advisors you will need are an attorney, an accountant, and a management consultant. You also will want a specialist in practice valuation if you are buying a practice. If you are joining a practice, you will need an attorney and an accountant. When working with more than one advisor, it is a good idea to have everyone meet together at least once to discuss your goals and coordinate their activities.

Selecting Advisors

Look for advisors who understand and have experience in health care. Recommendations from other physicians are a good starting point. Most national professional associations provide lists of their members. The American Medical Association has a national network of health care consultants and attorneys that have been screened. Your local medical society also may be able to provide referrals. Some medical societies provide legal help in employment contract negotiations and evaluating managed care contracts.

If you are starting your own practice, the three key advisors you will need are an attorney, an accountant, and a management consultant.

Before contacting a potential advisor, make a detailed list of the services you are looking for so you will be able to ask the advisor about specific experience in those areas. For example, if you are contacting attorneys regarding an employment contract, note the specific elements on which you would like advice, such as a recruitment incentive, partnership option, and restrictive covenant.

Listed as follows are criteria to consider in choosing any professional consultant:

- Experience working with physicians, especially obstetrician–gynecologists

- Positive recommendations from references provided (Box 3–1)

- Availability to you (eg, returns telephone calls promptly)

- Expertise in the specific areas in which you need help

- Philosophical compatibility with you in areas such as risk taking

- Personal rapport with you

- Membership in or certification by professional organization

- Cost

Ask a potential advisor to explain the services you can expect and estimate how long it will take. Find out exactly what information or documents the advisor will need from you to provide the services requested. Obtain specific information about any reports or documents the advisor will prepare, such as a business plan, policy manual, or financial statement. Expect your advisors to

---

BOX 3–1   CHECKING REFERENCES

Do not rely on written letters of recommendation because individuals will be more candid during a telephone call. You can ask the following questions:

- What services did the advisor provide for you?

- How satisfied were you with the service or advice provided?

- Would you use the advisor again? Why?

- What do you consider the consultant's strengths and weaknesses?

- How does this advisor compare with others you have used?

- Were the fees in line with your expectations?

---

specify, in writing, what services they will provide and what their fees are.

Attorneys

You should consult an attorney whenever you are considering an action with legal implications. These include signing an agreement, contracting with vendors, terminating an employee, or creating general or procedure specific informed consent forms.

Plan to interview several attorneys before making your decision. Prepare detailed questions about the topic on which you are seeking advice. An interview also gives you the opportunity to make sure you are comfortable personally. It is critical to have good rapport with your attorney.

You may want to interview attorneys from both small and large firms when making your selection. An advantage of using a large law firm is that it has the availability of attorneys who specialize in various aspects of law. You can select different attorneys for different legal issues, such as employment contracts or estate planning. The attorney you work with on your employment contract can confer with the tax expert, if needed. However, that extra consultation may cost you more.

With a small law firm or solo attorney, you can establish a relationship with a single attorney with a broad range of experience. You may prefer working with one individual for all your legal needs. Also, in comparison to being a client of a large firm that is handling huge corporate accounts, in a small firm you will be a relatively large account among its clients.

Fees

During your initial interview to select an attorney, you should discuss the fees and how they are structured. There may be a flat fee for routine tasks, such as filing corporate papers or preparing a simple will. Work rendered on projects that can require varying amounts of work, such as advising you on a contract or representing you in litigation, are most often charged by the hour. Rates vary with location and experience; lawyers in larger cities are likely to have higher fees than those in small towns.

If you are paying an attorney by the hour, you should receive an estimate of hours at the beginning of the arrangement, along with a description of services to be covered. For a specific project, you can ask for an hourly rate with a cap on the total amount. You should ask to be notified when the charges reach specific dollar amounts or a certain percentage of the total estimate.

A law firm also may have an annual retainer fee arrangement. Such arrangements can be useful if you have ongoing needs for legal services and want to establish an annual budget for them.

Whatever the arrangement, you should have a written fee agreement with your attorney. This agreement should clearly describe the scope of the representation and the method for calculating the fees.

Contract Advice

An important role of your attorney in any contract review is to be sure all aspects of the contract are legal. Your attorney also should advise you about what terms courts in your jurisdiction have found reasonable in past cases of disputes.

Employment Contract

When reviewing an employment contract, your attorney can help you in negotiations by framing the overall strategy as well as pointing out items that are not negotiable because of legal requirements. An attorney's experience with other physician employment contracts gives him or her valuable perspective on what are reasonable terms.

The attorney's advice about negotiating contract terms does not mean you must bring the attorney with you to negotiate. This is up to you. If you feel uncomfortable negotiating, your attorney can bring negotiating experience to the table. Be aware that if you do so, the group will do so as well. The presence of attorneys can add an adversarial flavor that can be counterproductive.

Managed Care Contracts

It is a good idea to have your attorney go over any managed care contract before you sign it. Legal scrutiny of any indemnification or hold harmless clauses, the availability of fee schedules, and the termination provisions are especially important.

Health Care and Business Law

In the highly regulated environment of medical practice, health law attorneys can help ensure that you meet legal and regulatory requirements. Health law attorneys make a point of staying abreast of current regulations so they can advise their clients when new regulations might affect them.

Some of the legal and regulatory issues that your attorney can help you with are as follows:

- Business licenses. Some locations require medical practices to obtain "business privilege" or "occupational" licenses to conduct the business of medicine. You also may need a zoning permit for your office.

- Clinical Laboratory Improvements Amendments requirements. An office laboratory must comply with the Clinical Laboratory Improvements Amendments. Many states also have their own laboratory requirements and require a state license.

- X-ray equipment license. State or local laws may govern the use and maintenance of X-ray equipment. An attorney should be consulted before installing such equipment; do not rely on the explanation of the equipment salesperson about the legal requirements.

- Private inurement. Tax-exempt entities are restricted from allowing their funds to be used to benefit individuals. Legal counsel can help you steer clear of any inurement pitfalls in your interactions with hospitals or other tax-exempt entities.

- Stark II legislation. Physicians are prohibited from referring Medicare or Medicaid patients to an entity providing health services (eg, radiology or physical therapy) if the physician has an ownership interest or compensation arrangement with the service. Any contract (including lease agreements) should be reviewed by an attorney competent in this area to ensure the terms comply with Stark II.

Chapter 10 gives more information on laws and regulations relevant to practice.

Other Legal Services

There are many other areas in which legal counsel can serve you, including:

- Office and equipment leases

- Personnel issues, such as firing an employee, review of personnel policy manual, and compliance with the Americans with Disabilities Act

- Will preparation and estate planning

- Medicare fraud and abuse issues

- Antitrust restrictions

Defense Attorneys

If you are named in a medical liability suit, your professional liability insurance carrier will assign an attorney to your case. Arrange a meeting with this attorney as soon as possible to discuss your case. Having a good rapport with your defense attorney is essential. If you do not feel comfortable with the assigned attorney, contact your insurance carrier and request new counsel. Most carriers will respect your wishes and try to accommodate you.

If your carrier's legal representation is not sufficient, that is, if you have been sued for more than the amount of coverage or your carrier is defending you under a "reservation of rights," you should retain your own defense counsel in addition to the carrier's attorney. Although your personal counsel might not lead the defense, he or she will be working exclusively for you and will represent your interests.

Evaluating a Defense Attorney

Consider the following criteria in assessing the insurance carrier's attorney or an attorney you retain to defend you:

- Competency—understanding the medicine involved

- Experience—handling of similar malpractice cases or claims

- Reputation—of the individual and the firm (ask your personal attorney to inquire)

- Approach to defense—sufficiently involving you in preparation

- Preparation—devoting adequate time and resources

- Rapport—you must be comfortable with and feel you can trust your attorney

- Conflict of interest—defense of other co-defendants

Defense Responsibilities

You have a role to play in your defense. You have the following responsibilities to your defense attorney:

- Make time for your attorney—litigation is a time-consuming process

- Never withhold any pertinent information

- Write a chronological summary of the incident

- Explain your treatment rationale, including alternative treatments

- Provide medical input, including relevant medical literature and identification of noted experts

- Go through your personal incident file with your attorney

- Ask questions and clear up any misunderstandings

- Learn the legal process; listen well—your attorney is the expert on litigation

Your defense attorney's responsibilities to you include:

- Keeping you informed about the litigation process

- Explaining the significance of each stage of the process

- Thoroughly preparing you for your role in each step

- Deciding the strategy and tactics of defense

- Ensuring that you are well prepared for any testimony you must give

Financial Advisors

An accountant or financial advisor can offer important counsel regarding the complex issues involved in compensation arrangements in a group medical practice. If you are seeking a loan for your practice, a financial advisor can help you prepare a business plan. Some experts point out that an accountant can be an "intangible asset" when borrowing money because the lender is impressed that you are approaching your practice professionally with advisors.

Selecting a Financial Advisor

Your financial advisor does not necessarily have to be a certified public accountant. Look for someone with the technical knowledge you need and with whom you have a good rapport.

Be sure your philosophy meshes with that of your accountant. In preparing tax returns, for example, there is a continuum of attitudes, from aggressive and willing to take risks with questionable deductions to conservative and unwilling to try anything that could conceivably be questioned. Most accountants' approaches fall somewhere in the middle of these two extremes.

Some practice management consultants have a great deal of financial expertise or accounting credentials. They may be able to provide accounting and tax services in addition to management consultation.

Types of Financial Advisors and Services

Personal Accountant

Listed as follows are examples of the areas in which a personal accountant can help you:

- Debt consolidation

- Developing a business plan

- Obtaining start-up capital

- Pay-out terms and tax implications of a signing bonus or recruitment incentive

- Tax implications of compensation packages, disability insurance benefits, retirement plans

- Terms of a buy-in agreement

- Tax return preparation

Bookkeeping and Accounting Services for Practice

Medical practices may retain an accounting service to handle accounting and tax matters for the practice. The service may do a minimal amount, such as prepare monthly or quarterly financial statements of income and disbursements, or they may provide extensive services. The following services are some that are available:

- Budget preparation

- Regular reports of accounts receivable and cash flow

- Training of office staff in bookkeeping procedures

- Establishing financial record systems and internal controls

- Routine audits

- Bank statement reconciliation

- Payroll management

Appraiser

Consult a professional with experience in practice appraisals to help you determine the value of a practice you are considering buying. The American Medical Association and obstetrician–gynecologists from other groups are good sources of references for appraisers. You should not consult with an appraiser who has a long-standing relationship with any of the parties involved in the buy-in. An objective outside party who is experienced at this type of appraisal should perform the valuation. The appraiser should be a member of one or more of the main professional associations for appraisers.

Medical Billing Services

Billing companies provide specific expertise in coding, working with third-party payers, collections, and fee schedules. Chapter 9 addresses the reimbursement process in more detail.

Practice Management Consultants

Some consultants charge a flat fee for specific services, but most charge by the hour. If you are starting your own practice, you will have the biggest need for management consultants. A 2004 article in *Medical Economics* noted that physicians should expect to pay a management consultant at least $5,000 during the start-up period and first year ("The First Steps, One Year Out," *Medical Economics*, March 19, 2004).

The following services are among those offered by practice consulting firms:

- Practice management. Consultants can provide expertise and guidance in staffing, billing services, equipment and supply needs, managed care contracts, and setting up systems for scheduling appointments.

- Facilities management. A firm can find office space and determine a layout for efficient patient flow.

- Financial management. Many practice management firms have accountants or financial experts on their staff who will provide services such as setting up bookkeeping and payroll systems. They also can provide advice on fee schedules.

- Information technology. Computer experts employed or retained by practice management firms will have experience in technology needs specific to medicine: appointment scheduling, Health Insurance Portability and Accountability Act compliant software, electronic medical records, billing software and electronic claims filing, as well as possibilities for electronic prescriptions and diagnostic orders.

Sources of Information

- The American College of Obstetricians and Gynecologists' "Practice Valuation: A Primer for Obstetrician–Gynecologists": www.acog.org or 800-673-8444

- American Medical Association ConsultingLink network: www.amaconsultinglink.com or 800-366-6968

- American Association of Healthcare Consultants: www.aahc.net or 888-350-2242

- American Bar Association: www.abanet.org or (312) 988-5000

- American Health Lawyers Association: www.healthlawyers.org or (202) 833-1100

- American Institute of Certified Public Accountants: www.aicpa.org or 888-777-7077

- American Society of Appraisers, Business Valuation Division: www.bvappraisers.org or (703) 478-2228

- Financial Planning Association: www.fpanet.org or 800-322-4237

- Institute of Certified Healthcare Business Consultants: www.ichbc.org or 800-447-1684

- Martindale-Hubbell's lawyer directory: www.martindale.com/xp/Martindale/home.xml

- Medical Group Management Association: www.mgma.com or 877-275-6462

- National Association of Healthcare Consultants: www.healthcon.org or 800-280-0750

- National CPA Health Care Advisors Association: www.hcaa.com or 800-869-0491

- National Healthcare Resource Center: 800-280-0750

- *Professional Liability and Risk Management: An Essential Guide for Obstetrician–Gynecologists*, published by the American College of Obstetricians and Gynecologists: sales.acog.org or 800-762-2264

- Society of Medical-Dental Management Consultants: www.smdmc.org or 800-826-2264

Chapter 4. Employment Contract Terms and Issues

Contract Basics

Get It in Writing

It may be true that some physicians join a practice on a handshake agreement, but this is not advisable. All terms guiding your relationship with the group should be explicit in a written agreement. Such agreements can take many forms, including a letter of an appointment or a formal contract; all are legally binding.

The following principles apply to all contracts:

- If the contract refers to other documents—bylaws, a health plan, or a retirement plan, for example—be sure you receive a copy of such documents, that they are dated, and that they are clearly identified in the agreement.

- Any exhibits or attachments to the contract are part of the contract and are enforceable.

- All parties to the contract must be named and must sign the agreement.

- Be sure you are given an original, signed contract for your files. (There can be multiple originals.)

- The contract should state provisions for renewing it and the process for amending it.

- The contract can identify the process for resolving major disagreements; such terms vary and may include binding arbitration or provisions that the prevailing party is reimbursed for legal fees and other costs.

All terms guiding your relationship with the group should be explicit in a written agreement.

What To Negotiate

Experts say that a common mistake physicians make in contract negotiations is accepting whatever is offered (see Chapter 7 for negotiating skills and strategies). Although a large practice with many employees has less leeway for making exceptions to its standard terms, in small practices, virtually everything is negotiable.

Do not try to negotiate on every point, however. Pick your battles by determining the issues that are most important to you, whether it is the expected workload, the compensation, the call schedule, or the options for partnership. Be firm on the issues that are most important to you and flexible on less critical areas.

Usually, you will do your own negotiating with the practice, consulting with your attorney or other advisors privately about the contract terms. If an impasse in the negotiations occurs, a strategy is to have your attorney negotiate for you. This sometimes works to distance you from problems caused by difficult negotiations.

TIP

If you are told that something in the contract is never enforced or will not ever apply to you, do not believe it. If it is in the contract, it is important.

Use Professional Advisors

Consult with an attorney familiar with the type of contract you are considering. The legality of some contract provisions can vary from state to state, so it is best to use a lawyer familiar with the jurisdiction where you will practice.

You should consult your accountant regarding specific aspects of contracts, such as the tax implications of compensation packages or of a bonus paid over a period of time. An accountant also can help you in structuring loans that may be part of the contract.

In buying a practice or signing a partnership contract involving a buy-in, you should work with an appraiser or consultant. The appraiser or consultant should be experienced in practice valuations.

Employee Agreement

Signing Bonus

A bonus for joining a practice is most common in areas that are underserved by physicians or locations that have drawbacks that make it difficult to recruit new physicians. If you are offered a bonus for joining the practice, find out why—it could be a red flag that there is a problem.

The contract should specify how you would be paid the bonus. A bonus is considered taxable income, so find out if taxes are to be withheld by the employer. The bonus may be paid to you over a period of time, with a provision that you pay back a prorated portion if you leave the practice within a given period.

A bonus also may be given as a loan against future income. The contract should spell out how the loan is to be paid back. You will want a clause that specifies that the loan will be forgiven in case of your death or disability.

Term

The term of a contract refers to how long it is in force before it expires or has to be renewed. For most new physicians, the term is 1 year, but it can be up to 3 years, depending on the practice. This initial term is considered a trial period for each party to assess the other, so the shortest period is in the best interest of both parties. If the practice wants you to be in a salaried, apprenticelike position for an extended period before you are offered partnership, this may be a red flag that the goal is to make money off you, not to add a colleague to the practice. Be sure the contract specifies the effective date.

Job Duties

Most contracts describe the conditions on which continued employment is contingent, such as appropriate licensure, maintaining hospital privileges, and participating in continuing medical education activities. It may include a requirement that you become board certified within a certain period. Other aspects of your work that the employment contract should cover are listed as follows:

- Responsibilities. Your job description should be clearly delineated in the agreement, including patient care responsibilities and administrative and teaching duties. Some contracts restrict physicians from doing certain procedures. Conversely, the practice may want you to provide special services that only you will perform. If this is the case, the contract should be specific about such services as well as the compensation and call schedule for them.

- Performance standards. The agreement should clarify how your performance will be evaluated and how the group handles peer review. The contract may include performance standards, utilization review, or cost-effectiveness; such performance assessments are more common with large groups and managed care organizations.

- Physician autonomy. Your clinical autonomy in treating patients as a licensed physician should be spelled out in the contract.

- Office hours. The contract should delineate office hours and how many hours per week you are expected to work. As a point of reference, the American College of Obstetricians and Gynecologists' survey of obstetric–gynecologic practices during 2003 reports that obstetrician–gynecologists in practice less than 5 years worked an average of 63 hours per week—50 hours in patient care and 13 hours in administration. (These reported hours do not include hours on-call.)

- Call coverage. Expectations for on-call hours should be spelled out. Try to eliminate vague wording, such as "reasonable call responsibilities." Call coverage responsibilities should be equitable among the physicians in the practice; that being said, seniority has its privileges, and it is not unusual for the newer members of the group to have more on-call hours than more established partners.

- Office space and resources. The sites where you are expected to practice (main office, satellite office, clinic) should be defined. In addition, the contract should cover the provision of clinical and office space and staff support adequate for you to carry out your duties.

- Outside activities. The contract may prohibit you from receiving compensation for services provided outside the practice. Examples of potentially restricted activities are moonlighting, teaching, and medical–legal consultation. If outside activites are permitted, the agreement should state whether you may retain all the income from such activities; some contracts specify that income from outside activities be distributed among all physicians in the practice.

Compensation

In comparing positions, consider the entire compensation package, not just the base salary. Some positions may guarantee a higher salary but require you to pay practice expenses. Fringe benefits and tax implications also change the compensation picture. In addition to defining the method of your compensation (eg, salary or salary-plus-productivity), the contract should cover the frequency of payment (such as every 2 weeks, monthly, or quarterly).

Straight Salary

A guaranteed straight salary for 1–2 years is common. If the agreement is for more than 1 year, it is customary for the salary to increase in the second or third year or for the contract to specify that a salary increase will be negotiated at certain intervals. Employment contracts sometimes cover options for receiving additional pay for extra hours worked.

Productivity Incentives

If you are offered a salary plus an incentive bonus, the contract should spell out the incentive and how it will be paid. A productivity bonus may be a percentage of the revenue you generate in excess of a set amount, such as two or three times your base salary. For example, if your base salary is $125,000, the productivity incentive may be a bonus of 20% of the revenue you generate over $250,000 or some other agreed-on amount. In contracts of more than 1 year where your base salary increases each year, the threshold amount for receiving a productivity bonus generally will increase as well.

The contract should be very clear about how productivity is defined, such as fees billed, hours worked, fees collected, or profits of the entire practice. The measures of productivity should cover details such as whether (and how) your productivity will be affected when you provide services to a partner's patients and vice-versa.

A productivity goal based on collected fees may be hard to reach, even if you are generating a lot of fees, because of the lag time for collections. This is especially relevant in obstetrics because services usually are billed after delivery.

TIP

Determine how you will be assigned patients and procedures. This area can be especially important if you have a productivity incentive based on patients seen or services billed.

Expenses

Expenses may be included in the compensation formula. If this is the case, the contract should specify how they are allocated.

Benefits

The benefits offered are as important in evaluating a position as the salary you will receive. In considering areas of the contract to negotiate, consider how important each benefit is to you.

Leave Time

A common (and minimal) arrangement for the first year is 2 weeks paid vacation and 1 week paid leave for continuing medical education. Paid sick days and parental leave time also should be specified. The contract should make clear the period of time specified for the designated leave time, such as 1 calendar year, 1 year from date of employment, or the practice's fiscal year.

Health Insurance

Health care insurance is an expensive benefit and, therefore, is an important element of the compensation plan. Be sure it covers your entire family.

Life Insurance

The practice may have a group life insurance policy for all the physicians with a death benefit. Premiums the group pays on insurance exceeding a $50,000 death benefit are considered taxable income to you by the Internal Revenue Service, so most small practices provide only the threshold of $50,000 of coverage.

Disability Insurance

Smaller groups are less likely to have a disability insurance plan in place than are large groups. If the practice pays premiums for your disability insurance, disability benefit payments are taxable when you receive them. Because of this tax disadvantage, you may want to negotiate to receive additional salary (equivalent to the disability insurance premium the practice would pay for you) and take out your own disability coverage; benefit payments would not then be taxed if you become disabled.

Medical Liability Insurance

Typically, your liability coverage will be paid by the group. If its policy is the claims-made type, your employment contract should specify who will pay for the insurance tail if you leave the group (see Chapter 6 for details about types of liability insurance). One contractual approach to handle this is to specify that the party that initiates the termination pays for the tail policy.

Retirement Plan

The employment contract should specify that you are eligible for the group's pension plan. The retirement plan benefits, such as the vesting schedule, are typically the same for all members of the group. The amount the group contributes to an employee's retirement usually is tied to the employee's total compensation.

Paid Expenses

Reimbursable expenses are benefits that sometimes can be negotiated if they are provided for the partners. These expenses may include cell phone or automobile expense to serve in a satellite office.

Professional Fees and Continuing Medical Education Allowance

Many practices pay for professional society dues, medical journal subscriptions, and hospital staff fees. The contract usually states a dollar limit for these items. A continuing medical education allowance with an annual cap ($2,000–$3,000) is common.

Moving Costs

Providing an allowance for your relocation is not universal, but many practices offer it. The amount can be negotiated. If the practice pays for your moving costs, the agreement will likely specify that you must reimburse the group if you leave voluntarily within a specified period.

Restrictive Covenant

A noncompete clause or "restrictive covenant" is included in most employment contracts, unless it is prohibited by state law. Most states allow restrictive covenants that are reasonable in scope and duration; check with your attorney or the state medical board about the law and how the courts have ruled in the practice's jurisdiction.

A noncompete clause prohibits you from practicing in the same area if you leave the group voluntarily. The clause will specify the geographic area and the period of time that are restricted. For example, you may be prohibited from practicing obstetrics and gynecology in certain counties or within a certain radius of the practice for the next 1 or 2 years.

The rationale behind a restrictive covenant is that the group has expended resources in recruiting you and setting you up in practice and does not want you to have the advantage of those resources if you leave the group and set up a competitive practice. In addition, you have knowledge of the group's business that could be useful in competition.

Sometimes the clause includes provisions for liquidated damages—an amount you would pay the employer if you do set up practice within the restricted area and time period. What is a reasonable amount for liquidated damages varies; some contracts set damages at an amount equal to 1 year's base salary. The amount should not be determined as a penalty but as a reasonable estimate of the economic loss the practice would incur by your establishing a competitive practice.

There may be only one other physician in the practice. In this case, the contract usually states that the restrictive covenant is dissolved in the event of that physician's death.

You and your attorney should review any noncompete language carefully and try to limit the restrictions. The restrictive covenant is an area in which both you and the practice have legitimate but conflicting concerns. Usually, the terms can be negotiated to reach a satisfactory compromise that is reasonable and fair for both parties.

Listed as follows are negotiating points that might mitigate the effects of a noncompete clause:

- If the group has multiple offices, restrictions that apply to all satellite locations would be considered severe.

- If your employment is terminated (except for cause) or if you are not offered a partner position at the end of the contract term, the noncompete clause does not go into effect.

- A grace period—an initial period such as 6 months—is established before the restrictive covenant goes into effect. The rationale for a grace period is that in such a short period you would not have garnered enough patients to be a competitive threat to the practice.

TIP

Beware of restrictive covenant provisions that include a hospital that would be important to your practice.

Termination

Your agreement should include a section describing the conditions under which your employment contract can be terminated. There are two basic types of termination:

1. For cause. The contract may have a section describing circumstances under which you could be terminated "for cause" or for "just

cause." Conditions warranting termination for cause are typically serious lapses, and termination usually is immediate. Examples of conditions of termination for just cause are loss of medical license, use of illegal drugs, or conviction of a felony. It is important the contract clearly defines "cause," and you should try to have it defined as narrowly as possible. Beware of subjective language, such as "inappropriate behavior" or "actions that are negative to the practice."

2. Termination with notice. The contract may state that employment is "at will," which means that either party may end the employment at any time without specifying a reason by giving sufficient written notice. Notice can vary from 30 to 120 days, during which time you continue to work and receive a salary and fringe benefits.

The termination section also may address the ownership of medical records. Usually the practice retains the ownership of the records of the patients you treat.

Future Partnership

The contract may cover the conditions under which you can become a partner or stockholder in the group. An alternative is a detailed letter of intent in addition to the initial employment contract.

If you are interested in becoming a partner, be sure the language, whether in the contract or a separate document, states specific conditions, not vague criteria that will make you eligible for partnership. Avoid language that states the group has an "intent" of offering partnership or promises that consideration of your partnership will be "reviewed" or "discussed" at a certain time. The contract or letter of intent also should state what will happen if another physician in the group dies or becomes disabled before you gain full partnership.

Partnership or Shareholder Agreement

Buy-In

In many practices, to become a partner you must buy in to a practice by paying an agreed-on amount to the other partners. If the amount of a buy-in has been previously set for all new partners, you may have little room for negotiation. Nevertheless, you should ask for a description of how the valuation was done.

The structure of the buy-in is a critical part of the partnership arrangement. This amount usually is based on the value of the business, which can be calculated using many different formulas. Part of the buy-in price may be a determination of the value of tangible assets, such as property and equipment, less the practice debt. The value of the accounts receivable may be another component of the valuation. If the amount of accounts receivable is used, be sure your own contributions to the receivables are not included.

The following key points should be clarified:

- Will your percentage of ownership be the same as that of the other partners?

- Will your ownership include a percentage of the facility, equipment, supplies, and accounts receivable?

- If accounts receivable are used as part of the buy-in calculation, do they reflect the normal and expected pattern of income?

If you are paying the amount of the buy-in over a period of time, the agreement should specify the interest rate and frequency and duration of your payments. Consult your accountant about the tax implications of your payback arrangement.

Some groups allow you to buy in to the practice using "sweat equity." In this type of buy-in arrangement, rather than paying a dollar amount, you have responsibility for certain activities, such as extra call coverage.

Decision-Making Authority

The contract should state whether you will have an equal voice with the other partners in making decisions affecting the practice. A large practice may have an established governance structure with officers or committees with assigned responsibilities for making decisions, such as office policies and fees, staffing, hiring and firing physicians, and participation in managed care contracts. In smaller groups, such decisions may be voted on by all partners.

Income Distribution

Groups use different methods for distributing income among partners. Some distribute income equally, some use productivity measurements, and some use a formula that combines productivity and other factors. Productivity can be calculated using numerous measures, such as how much revenue you generate, how many hours you work, or how many patients you see.

Sometimes the group gives weight to other factors in determining remuneration by assigning points to variables such as:

- Seniority
- Board certification or special training
- Administrative duties
- New patients
- Use of equipment
- Research or teaching activities

The partnership contract should spell out the method used for income distribution and the factors used in the productivity formula, if applicable.

Expense Allocation

How the practice allocates expenses to each partner is another important element of income that should be addressed in the partnership agreement. The following accounting methods may be in place for allocation of expenses:

- Equal assessment. The total for expenses is subtracted from the gross revenue before the income is distributed among the partners. This works best when all physicians have approximately equal schedules and responsibilities.

- Direct cost allocation. The costs incurred by each physician are charged directly to that physician. This approach accommodates the use of equipment and staff not used by all the partners.

- Indirect cost allocation. Fixed overhead costs, such as those for rent and utilities, are charged to each physician, usually as a per-square-foot charge.

- Allocation based on time worked. This method can be used to accommodate physicians who work part-time.

- Allocation as percentage of productivity. The percentage of expenses charged to each physician equals the percentage of revenue generated. Thus, an obstetrician–gynecologist who generates 30% of the income will be charged 30% of the expenses.

Partnership Termination and Buy-Out

The contract should specify how your ownership interest can be transferred or terminated. Circumstances that could call for such a transaction include your voluntary or involuntary termination, death, disability, retirement, divorce, or bankruptcy. The agreement should make clear how the amount of your buy-out (your equity) would be calculated, the length of time for you to be paid in full if you are bought out, and the interest to be paid on the balance due. In addition, the fate of shared assets, including equipment and real estate, should be spelled out. The contract also may state circumstances under which the amount of the buy-out would be decreased or the buy-out might be eliminated, such as if you establish a practice in competition with the group.

Sources of Information

- *Buy-In Agreements,* published by the Medical Group Management Association (includes descriptions and samples of buy-in agreements from 500 groups surveyed): www.mgma.com

- *Buying, Selling, and Owning the Medical Practice, 2nd Edition*, published by the American Medical Association (AMA): www.amapress.com or 800-621-8335

- *Evaluating and Negotiating Your Compensation Arrangements*, published by the AMA: www.amapress.com or 800-621-8335

- *The Legal Basis of Medical Practice— MPM's Guide*, published by the *Journal of Medical Practice Management* (has helpful guides to employment agreements and how to evaluate them): www.mpmnetwork.com or 800-933-3711

- *Physician Compensation and Production Survey*, published annually by the Medical Group Management Association (reports survey results for both academic and private practice; it costs several hundred dollars, so check your medical or hospital library): www.mgma.com or 877-275-6462

- Physician Model Employment Agreement, prepared by the AMA. Accessible to AMA members only at www.ama-assn.org

- *Practice Patterns of Obstetrics/Gynecology, 2003*, published by the AMA (reports data from 2001–02 survey on obstetric–gynecologic revenue, expenses, weeks worked, and hospital utilization): www.amapress.com or 800-621-8335

- *Profile of Ob-Gyn Practice*, published by the American College of Obstetricians and Gynecologists (reports 2003 survey data on obstetric–gynecologic average hours worked, procedures, patient visits): www.acog.org or 800-673-8444

Chapter 5. **Licensing and Credentialing**

Getting a state medical license and hospital privileges in a new location can be a rigorous and time-consuming process, so you should start the process at least 6 months before you plan to practice. Once you know where you will practice, begin applying for the licenses and credentials you will need.

State Licensure

You must obtain a medical license in each state in which you practice. The web site of the Federation of State Medical Boards (www.fsmb.org) has links to each state medical board's web site. You can check online for licensing information and download application forms or call the state medical board for an application packet.

Plan on 2–4 months after you submit your application for the process to be complete, but it can drag out to 6 months if there are problems. If you graduated from a medical school outside the United States, expect it to take longer.

If you have less-than-positive information in your medical background, such as a disciplinary action, openly disclose this when you submit your application, help the licensing board obtain any necessary records, and explain any mitigating circumstances. These steps will facilitate the entire process and help foreclose a potential denial of licensure.

The Federation of State Medical Boards has established the Federation Credentials Verification Service (FCVS) to store and verify information that is required to obtain a medical license. If you set up an FCVS portfolio, FCVS stores the data for the rest of your life and verifies it for any state medical board to which you apply. This can be very helpful if you apply for licensure in more than one state or think you might move to another state in the future. Some state licensing boards require an FCVS physician profile when you apply for a license in that state.

The Federation Credentials Verification Service charges an initial fee ($275 in 2004) to create your portfolio. Once the profile is set

You must obtain a medical license in each state in which you practice.

up, there is no annual charge to maintain it, but there is a fee ($45–$65 in 2004) each time you have it sent to a new entity.

Drug Enforcement Administration Registration

The Drug Enforcement Administration (DEA) web site (www.dea.gov) has forms, instructions, and information you will need to register for a license to prescribe drugs. New DEA applications are processed within 4–6 weeks.

Some states require their own narcotics license in addition to that of the DEA. The application process for both the DEA and state registration has been coordinated so you can complete applications for both when applying for your DEA registration.

National Provider Identifier

The Centers for Medicare & Medicaid Services is in the process of establishing a universal identifier for each physician. Every physician will be assigned a 10-digit number called the National Provider Identifier (NPI).

The Centers for Medicare & Medicaid Services will begin distributing NPIs in May 2005. If you have participated in Medicare, you will automatically receive your new NPI, which will replace the unique physician identification number previously used for Medicare providers. If you do not already have a unique physician identification

number, you can apply for an NPI after May 23, 2005. The Centers for Medicare & Medicaid Services web site (www.cms.hhs.gov) gives details about the application process.

All insurers—both public and private—will eventually be required to use NPIs. The NPI will replace the many separate numbers that different insurance plans have used for provider reimbursement. The NPI system was mandated by the Health Insurance Portability and Accountability Act and is intended to improve the efficiency of the health care system.

All insurers except small health plans must start using NPIs by May 23, 2007. The compliance date for small health plans is May 23, 2008.

Hospital Credentialing

Obtaining hospital privileges can be a tedious process. Try to keep in mind that the purpose of the application and approval process is not to make you jump through hoops but to ensure that patients receive good care.

A hospital uses the credentialing process to verify that you are qualified to perform specific procedures, can work effectively with colleagues and hospital staff, and will abide by the hospital's rules and regulations. You may have to pay a fee to the hospital to process your application.

Most hospitals require the following documentation when you apply for staff privileges:

• Personal information, including previous addresses

• Medical education and training records (copies of diplomas)

• Employment history, including job descriptions and references for each job

• Current and past hospital affiliations

• References regarding competence, judgment, and character

• Lists of procedures you have done and for which you seek privileges

• Current and past state licensure

- Drug Enforcement Administration registration

- Military service

- Membership in medical associations

- Certificate of medical liability insurance coverage

- Proof of board certification(s)

- List of continuing medical education activities

- Previous liability claims, challenges to licensure, or loss of privileges at another hospital

The following steps are typical in obtaining medical staff privileges:

1. The hospital staff verifies the accuracy of the information you provided.

2. The credentials committee evaluates your application; in some cases, an interview with the committee is part of the process. The credentials committee makes a recommendation to the medical staff executive committee.

3. The executive committee considers your application and makes a recommendation to the hospital's board of trustees.

4. After consideration of the executive committee's recommendation, the board of trustees grants or denies medical staff membership.

If you are denied privileges to practice at a hospital, check the medical staff bylaws to find out the appeals process.

Delineation of Privileges

Part of your application for medical staff membership will be a "Delineation of Privileges" form from the obstetric–gynecologic department listing clinical procedures. These often are grouped into Levels I, II, and III. Level I comprises the most basic or core procedures, and each successive level includes the procedures of the lower level.

When you indicate the clinical privileges you are requesting, you must submit evidence of your competence to perform them. Such evidence may be a list of the procedures you performed in training. You may be asked to provide case information, including patient history, physical examination, and discharge summary.

Evaluation and Verification of Your Application

Hospital staff do not begin to check your references and verify your education and licensure until all the required materials have been received. The hospital staff will verify virtually all the information you provide by contacting the source, such as the state medical board; your undergraduate, graduate, and medical schools; the institution where you completed residency; and individuals who have furnished reference letters. You should expect the obstetric–gynecologic department chair to interview you to discuss your application for clinical privileges.

Hospitals are required to query the National Practitioner Data Bank, both when you apply and every 2 years after that. In addition, the hospital may query the Healthcare Integrity and Protection Data Bank and the Federal Physician Data Center (Box 5–1).

A record of an adverse action in one of these data banks does not mean that your request for privileges will automatically be rejected. Be sure you report in advance any such actions that have become a part of your record, rather than omitting this information from your application. It is better to acknowledge the action and provide a written explanation at the start of the application process. The credentials committee has a duty to investigate such reports and will require a satisfactory explanation of any adverse actions in your file.

Follow-up Is Critical

After you submit your application to the hospital, the staff will contact you if they are missing any required materials. You should provide the missing information as quickly as possible. The hospital will not begin the verification process until all the documentation is received.

BOX 5–1 PHYSICIAN DATA BANKS

Hospitals and other eligible organizations are entitled to query the following data banks that maintain physician information:

- National Practitioner Data Bank. Established by the Health Care Quality Improvement Act of 1986 as a central repository of information on physicians, dentists, and other health care practitioners, this data bank contains information on medical liability payments and any adverse actions against your licensure, clinical privileges, and professional society memberships.

- Healthcare Integrity and Protection Data Bank. This data bank was established as part of the Health Insurance Portability and Accountability Act of 1996. Designed to combat fraud and abuse in health delivery and reimbursement, it reports final adverse actions taken against health care providers.

- Federation Physician Data Center. Maintained by the Federation of State Medical Boards specifically for the credentials verification process, this source has data on disciplinary actions against physicians by state and international licensing boards. This data bank may be accessed only by organizations entitled to verify credentials, but the Federation of State Medical Boards also provides a data bank of disciplinary actions for public access at www.docinfo.org.

Check with the hospital credentialing staff periodically to be sure everything is in order. The staff could be waiting for a missing item, while you are assuming that the process is going forward. This delay could lead to your having to submit updated information and begin the process again.

Types of Hospital Privileges

Hospitals have several categories of membership for which privileges are granted. Your medical staff rights and responsibilities, such as voting, holding office, attending meetings, and providing emergency call coverage, will vary according to the type of privileges you are granted.

Listed as follows are the typical types of hospital privileges:

- Temporary. If your medical staff application is not complete and you need to provide call coverage in your group, the hospital may be willing to issue you temporary privileges.

- Probationary. This is the category usually granted to newly privileged physicians.

- Courtesy. Physicians may seek courtesy privileges when they want to maintain the ability to practice in the hospital but rarely admit or attend patients there.

- Active or attending. These privileges are granted when you have passed the probationary period. You might be required to admit a minimum number of patients per year to retain active privileges on the medical staff.

TIP

Read the medical staff bylaws to find out the requirements for maintaining privileges at the hospital.

Outcome

You may be granted the privileges you requested or given a medical staff appointment somewhat different from the one you requested. If you are denied privileges, you will likely have recourse to an appeal process.

Usually, you will initially be given probationary privileges. During the probationary period, a physician may oversee your performance regarding competent technique, compliance with required documentation, and adherence to hospital policy and procedures. This supervising physician will evaluate your performance at the end of your probationary period.

Following this evaluation, you will 1) be granted full privileges, 2) be required to hone certain clinical skills before receiving full privileges, or 3) receive "modified acceptance" of your application. Modified acceptance usually means that certain requested procedures are excluded from your privileges, perhaps contingent on additional training and supervision in those areas.

If you are denied privileges for more than 30 days because of incompetence or unprofessional conduct, this denial must be reported to the

National Practitioner Data Bank. However, a denial or restriction is not reported if your privileges are denied or restricted solely because you do not meet the hospital's threshold eligibility criteria for a particular privilege.

Economic Credentialing

Competition for patients has led some hospitals to use referral patterns of physicians as part of their decision to grant privileges. This is called "economic credentialing," which the American Medical Association (AMA) defines as "the use of economic criteria unrelated to quality of care or professional competence in determining a physician's qualifications for initial or continuing hospital medical staff membership or privileges." Some hospitals have established conflict-of-interest policies or loyalty oaths and refuse to grant staff privileges to physicians who admit patients to competing health care entities or who have financial interests or leadership positions with other health care organizations.

The AMA opposes economic credentialing and encourages medical staff members to work with a hospital's governing body to resolve such issues and to develop appropriate conflict-of-interest policies. If you encounter an obstacle to credentialing that seems unrelated to the quality of patient care, contact the AMA Department of Organized Medical Staff Services at (312) 464-4761 or www.ama-assn.org/go/omss.

Managed Care Credentialing

A managed care organization will not add you to its panel of approved providers until you complete its credentialing process. The credentialing process for managed care plans is similar to that used in hospitals, with the following differences:

- Credentialing is governed by a contract rather than a governing body, such as the hospital board of trustees.

- The objective is to join a network or panel of providers.

- The process will include a site visit to your office.

- For physicians with practice experience, managed care plans also may evaluate the efficiency of patient care using criteria such as length of stay and hospitalization costs.

To eliminate the duplication of effort in applying to different hospitals and health care organizations, a number of organizations, both commercial and nonprofit, have developed standardized applications for physicians to use. For example, a standardized process was launched in 2003 by a nonprofit coalition of the largest managed care plans—the Council for Affordable Quality Healthcare (CAQH). In the CAQH universal system, which is a free service, you fill out one application online and update it or confirm that it is accurate every 3 months after that. By mid 2004, 40 health plans were participating in the CAQH system, including some of the largest.

Another example of a uniform application process is the Integrated Massachusetts Application for Initial Credentialing, which was created under the auspices of the Massachusetts Medical Society in 2004. Major health plans in the state collaborated on a uniform application that physicians can use with seven different health plans.

Check for available uniform credentialing applications when you apply to participate with a managed care organization. The organization may use an application you have already completed.

TIP

Get the name and telephone number of the provider relations staff for each payer; follow-up with that individual until your application is approved.

Sources of Information

- American Medical Association Department of Organized Medical Staff Services: www.ama-assn.org/go/omss or (312) 464-4761

- Centers for Medicare & Medicaid Services: www.cms.hhs.gov

- Council for Affordable Quality Healthcare: www.caqh.org or 888-599-1771

- *Credentialing, Privileging, Competency, and Peer Review: Examples of Compliance for the Medical Staff,* published in 2003 by Joint Commission Resources: www.jcrinc.com/publications or 877-223-6866

- Drug Enforcement Administration: www.dea.gov or 800-882-9539

- Federation Credentials Verification Service: www.fsmb.org or 888-275-3287

- Federation Physician Data Center: www.drdata.org or (817) 868-4072; public version at www.docinfo.org

- Federation of State Medical Boards: www.fsmb.org or (817) 868-4000

- *State Medical Licensure Requirements and Statistics 2005,* published by the AMA: www.amapress.com or 800-621-8335

- U.S. Medical Licensing Examination: www.usmle.org or (215) 590-9600

Chapter 6.   Insurance

Professional Liability Insurance

You should be familiar with the terms of your professional liability insurance coverage even if you are not purchasing the policy yourself. If your group is buying your insurance or you are a resident or fellow in training, use the information in this section as a guide to find out the details of the coverage you have.

Always obtain and keep a copy of the policy for each year of your coverage during both training and practice. Years later you could be named in a lawsuit for that period, and the carrier is not obligated to retain a record of your coverage. The policy itself is the best proof that you were insured. You also should keep copies of all your communications with the carrier.

Types of Policies

Professional liability insurance comes in two basic forms: 1) occurrence or 2) claims-made. In some areas, only claims-made policies are available. In the 2003 ACOG Survey on Professional Liability, the following percentages of obstetrician–gynecologists responding reported having the following types of professional liability insurance: 24.3% occurrence, 52%, claims-made, 4.1% other, 0.3% self-insured, and 19.3% do not know or no answer.

Occurrence Policies

Occurrence coverage provides lifetime coverage for incidents that occurred while the policy was in effect, regardless of when the claim is filed. Thus, if you have an occurrence-type policy in effect for the calendar year 2005 and a patient files a claim in 2010 for an incident that happened during 2005, the policy covers you for that claim, even if you no longer have insurance with that carrier.

> *You should be familiar with the terms of your professional liability insurance coverage even if you are not purchasing the policy yourself.*

The premiums for occurrence insurance are typically higher than those for claims-made policies. When a claim is filed, the limits for the claim are what were specified when the policy was in effect for that period. An occurrence policy does not cover claims for incidents that happened before you had the policy.

TIP

Occurrence policies are good for obstetrician–gynecologists because a claim for an impaired infant might be filed years after the event happened.

Claims-Made Policies

Claims-made insurance provides coverage only for incidents that occurred and were reported while you are insured with that carrier. Thus, both the incident and the filing of the claim must happen while the policy is in effect. If you are sued the day after you drop a claims-made policy (eg, by changing to another carrier when you move or join a new group practice, for example), you would not be covered, even if the incident occurred during the period the policy was in effect unless you purchased "tail coverage."

An extended reporting endorsement—an additional policy known as tail coverage—is needed to cover you after a claims-made policy ends. This additional policy for tail coverage is expensive; a ballpark estimate is one-and-a-half to three times the regular annual premium. Tail coverage is essential, however, so you will be insured against liability for any claims that arise from incidents that occurred during the effective period of the policy.

An alternative to tail coverage is "nose" coverage or "prior acts coverage," which you may be able to purchase from your new liability carrier. If you are changing carriers, ask your new carrier for a quote for prior acts coverage and compare it with the cost of buying tail coverage from your old insurance carrier.

When you purchase tail or prior acts coverage, be sure the retroactive date covers the period of your previous claims-made policy. Also, clarify the terms of coverage, including the aggregate limit. The aggregate limit is the total amount of money the policy will pay for all claims combined. Sometimes the aggregate limit in tail insurance applies to the entire period the policy is in effect rather than a single year.

Claims-Paid Policies

A variation on claims-made coverage is a claims-paid policy, which is the least expensive type of professional liability coverage. With claims-paid coverage, all the events associated with a claim—the incident, the filing of a lawsuit, and the final resolution or settlement of the claim—must occur during the period the policy is in place. The policy will not cover you if any of those events occurs outside the effective dates of the policy. Thus, although claims-paid coverage is inexpensive, it is risky.

TIP

If you leave a practice that agreed to pay for tail coverage for you on departure, verify directly with the carrier that the required payment was received.

Coverage

Most policies offer limits of coverage ranging from $100,000/$300,000 to $1 million/$3 million. The first number is the maximum the insurance company will pay per claim during the policy period, which usually is 12 months. The second amount is the maximum the company will pay for all claims during the policy period.

In the 2003 ACOG Survey on Professional Liability, the average professional liability coverage reported by obstetrician–gynecologists was for limits of $1 million/$3 million. Many hospitals require $1 million/$3 million limits for staff privileges.

Be sure the limits of your coverage are adequate for an obstetric–gynecologic practice in your area. In states with caps on damages, you may not need limits as high as elsewhere.

You will be personally responsible for paying any damages that exceed your coverage limits. Chapter 12 provides strategies for you to protect your assets in case a judgment against you is higher than the limits of your insurance coverage.

In addition to the limits, the policy will specify what incidents are covered. Be sure the insurance covers your full scope of clinical activities. Verify that the coverage applies to your professional corporation and employees. Determine if these limits are shared by all or apply to each individual.

If you are in solo practice or a small practice, you may want your policy to include insurance for locum tenens coverage. Many policies include such coverage for 30–120 days annually, with no additional premium.

Premiums

Insurance carriers operate on the principle of spreading risk among those whom they insure. Carriers use the premiums paid by policy holders to build reserves necessary to pay losses from claims and lawsuits, to cover the expenses of operating the company, and to guarantee future solvency.

The following factors may be used by some carriers to determine the amount of a premium:

- The outcomes and settlement amounts of any past claims against you (known as "experience rating")

- Your specialty, certification, and years of practice experience

- The location of your practice

Although inexpensive premiums are nice, be wary if an insurer's rates seem abnormally low compared to those of other companies. Claims-made policies are cheaper than occurrence policies for the first several years of coverage because the potential for claims builds slowly as policy years accumulate. Premiums for claims-made policies increase each year for a period, such as 5 years, until they reach what is called the "mature rate." The first-year premium may be very inexpensive, such as 30% of the mature rate. Be sure to ask how much the premium will increase after the first year; the second-year premium may be twice as much.

Some policies have variable premiums depending on a deductible amount that you must pay before the insurer pays for costs, awards, or settlements that exceed the deductible. Be sure to consider the deductible when comparing premium rates.

For claims-made policies, some carriers offer free tail coverage on retirement, death, or disability if you have been a policy holder for several years—usually 5 years or more. Check to see if your carrier offers a reduced premium if you participate in specified risk-management education or if you do not have any claims for a certain period.

TIP

You can lower your premiums by choosing a higher deductible.

Defense Costs

Check on the policy's coverage of defense costs, which are the expenses involved in defending and processing a suit—not the amount of the award or settlement. Defense costs include the fees of the defense attorney retained by the insurance company, the fees of expert witnesses, court reporters' fees, and clerical expenses.

Some policies do not pay for defense costs or put a limit on the amount the insurance company will pay. If your policy does cap the amount of defense costs it will cover, be sure the overall policy limit is high enough to cover defense costs in addition to a settlement or judgment amount. This means that coverage should be for "ultimate net loss" instead of "pure loss." Ultimate net loss coverage pays for attorney fees and defense costs in addition to any awards.

If you are sued for more than the amount of coverage or your carrier is defending you under a "reservation of rights," you should consider retaining your own defense counsel in addition to the carrier's attorney. Having ultimate net loss coverage may allow you to recover expenses you have if you retain your own defense attorney.

Remember that any written or recorded information you give to the insurer is subject to discovery. As soon as a defense attorney is assigned to your case, you should communicate exclusively with him or her about the case; such communications will be protected by attorney-client privilege (see Chapter 3 for more details about how to work with your defense attorney).

Policy Exclusions

Every medical liability insurance policy has an exclusions section. An exclusions section details specific circumstances under which coverage will not apply.

Hold-Harmless Exclusion

Many medical liability insurance policies exclude coverage for liability that a physician assumes by contract. However, many managed care contracts require you to hold the organization harmless if it is sued by a patient in connection with your performance of services. Thus, if you agree to a hold-harmless clause with a managed care plan, you could end up having no liability coverage if a patient enrolled in the managed care plan sues the managed care organization. You might have to assume liability for your own and the managed care plan's defense costs as well as any judgment or settlement. Ask your insurer whether you will be protected if you sign a hold-harmless clause or whether this restriction can be waived. Your medical liability policy may not use the term "hold harmless" in its exclusion section, so you should carefully scrutinize the exclusions section for any exclusion to coverage.

Vicarious Liability Exclusion

A policy also may exclude coverage for vicarious liability, which could include liability arising from the actions of your employees. For example, if a staff member's labeling error results in treatment that harms a patient, you could be sued for the employee's error. If your policy excludes vicarious liability, you may be liable for the defense costs and judgment of the lawsuit. Some policies have variations regarding exclusions for vicarious liability. For example, your policy may exclude only vicarious actions of employees who are allied health practitioners.

If you are a partner in a group practice that is chartered or incorporated, each partner's individual insurance policy should provide coverage for vicarious liability. Such coverage protects all the partners in the event of a large settlement or judgment.

You may be able to negotiate with your insurer to add coverage for vicarious liability for an additional premium. Examine your policy carefully to ascertain who in your practice is not covered and purchase vicarious liability coverage if necessary.

Mandated Standards of Care

Some policies require you to adhere to certain standards to maintain your liability coverage. For example, liability during surgery may be covered only if a board-certified anesthesiologist administers anesthesia, or coverage may apply only if you use certain equipment in practice.

Be aware of the policy's mandated standards of care before you purchase the insurance. Be sure that any mandated standards of care in your policy do not restrict your practice style or significantly increase overhead expenses.

Other Common Exclusions

Claims involving the following factors also may be excluded from coverage:

- Sexual misconduct
- Practicing under the influence of alcohol or illegal drugs
- Antitrust violations
- Criminal or grossly negligent acts
- Libel, slander, or invasion of privacy
- Procedures for which you have not received credentials
- Newly developed or experimental procedures
- Restraint of trade because of peer-review or quality-assurance activities
- Use of drugs still under Investigational New Drug status or not yet approved by the U.S. Food and Drug Administration or both

In addition, coverage usually is excluded for lawsuits that arise from incidents that include violations of patient confidentiality, failure of medical devices, or inadequate quality control of medications. Finally, injuries that do not involve patient care, such as those resulting from a fall in your reception area, often are excluded. Alternatively, some policies include "premise liability" coverage for such injuries as an "extra bonus," but this extra coverage will likely duplicate coverage you are paying for in your property liability insurance.

Consent-to-Settle Clauses

A settlement is an agreement made between the parties to a lawsuit or claim that resolves their dispute. Any payment made on your behalf by an insurance company must be reported to the National Practitioner Data Bank. Thus, any such settlement can adversely affect your insurance status, ability to participate in a managed-care group, and application for hospital privileges.

Check to see if your insurance policy contains a clause specifying that no case will be settled without the physician's written consent. If your policy does not have a "consent-to-settle" clause, the insurer can settle a case against your wishes, even if you are blameless. If the policy grants you this right, you must be consulted before any settlement offers or counteroffers are made. This is something you want and should try to negotiate to be included.

Nevertheless, you should be aware that there can be good reasons to settle a claim. A settlement could allow you to avoid a verdict that exceeds your insurance coverage. Another reason you may wish to settle is to avoid spending additional time, energy, and money on the litigation process. The attorney assigned to your case should inform you of the choices, the risks with each approach, and the alternatives that are available. Disagreements between the physician and the insurer concerning a settlement are sometimes referred to a committee for resolution.

Some policies have what is called a "hammer clause" instead of a consent-to-settlement clause. The terms of a hammer clause take effect if you refuse the insurer's settlement recommendation and choose to go to trial instead. Then, if the trial results in an award higher than the settlement recommendation, you must pay the amount that is more than the recommendation. Before you purchase a policy, try to negotiate the terms so that your policy includes a consent-to-settlement clause and omits a hammer clause.

Other Policy Elements To Examine

In addition to coverage, defense costs, exclusions, and settlement rights, be sure you understand the specifics about the following aspects of your professional liability policy:

- Reporting requirements. The policy may state that you must report a bad outcome, a liability claim, or a request for information from a patient's lawyer "promptly" or "within a reasonable time." Find out what is considered reasonable and what happens if a claim is not reported within that period.

- Disclosure requirements. Policies usually have requirements for "full disclosure." Find out the definition of "full" and what the implications are for failure to provide full disclosure.

- Claims processing. Check the company's procedures for handling claims. Ask about the experience of the claims staff and whether they handle only medical malpractice claims. Find out how much you will be involved in case review and in resolving a claim.

- Defense policies. Determine the extent of the insurer's obligation to defend you, including whether you will be compensated for time away from practice. Clarify what happens if a claim has multiple defendants.

What To Look for in a Carrier

Before signing an insurance policy, investigate the insurance company's background, reputation, and services. Your state insurance commissioner's office can provide information about insurers licensed in your state. A license indicates the insurer has met the state's minimum standards and is authorized to sell the lines of insurance for which it is licensed. State insurance departments also may be permitted to give information about complaints that have been filed against the insurer.

The American College of Obstetricians and Gynecologists' Department of Professional Liability and the Physician Insurers Association of America can provide helpful information about insurance companies. Local hospitals and your state medical society also are good resources for information about insurance companies.

Check out the carrier's A.M. Best rating; it should be "A" or "A Excellent." A.M. Best Company is an independent industry analyst that rates property and casualty insurance carriers in its annual *A.M. Best's Insurance Reports— Property and Casualty*. You can find it in public libraries or through your insurance agent. Other insurance rating services also can provide information about the stability of a carrier.

It is a good idea to talk to a physician who has experienced a claim with the carrier. Find out how the claim was handled, how much the physician was involved in resolving the claim, and whether he or she was satisfied with the carrier's handling of it.

You should ask whether the carrier has risk management programs for physicians. You also should find out whether a program is in place to provide emotional support for defendants.

TIP

Look for an agent with experience in medical liability insurance, not just in general liability insurance.

Types of Insurance Carriers

There are many types of insurance carriers. Insurers vary in how they are organized, who owns or controls them, their financial stability, and whether and how they are regulated by state laws.

Commercial Carriers

Commercial insurance carriers are regulated by state insurance departments and may provide coverage nationwide or at least in numerous states. These companies must meet state requirements and usually are backed by state guaranty funds. Guaranty funds are funds established by law in every state to protect policy holders if an insur-

ance carrier faces financial insolvency or is unable to meet its financial obligations.

An advantage of commercial carriers is their financial stability. Large companies may offer both professional liability insurance and business-owners coverage and give you a discount if you purchase both types. Also, for multistate companies, you can continue your coverage if you move to another state. A drawback of commercial carriers is that, as for-profit organizations with the goal of making a profit for their stockholders, they may pull out of a market if it becomes unprofitable.

Captive Companies

A captive insurance company is a wholly-owned subsidiary of an association or group, such as a university hospital or a medical society. Unlike a commercial carrier, a captive company is formed with the express purpose of insuring the members of the association or group that has formed it.

Captive companies typically are not protected by state guaranty funds. They are nonprofit entities that base their insurance premiums on the claims history of the insureds and actual expenses instead of on market fluctuations.

An advantage of a captive company is that it is owned and directed by health care professionals, who are more likely to understand and be supportive of your professional problems than are the managers of commercial carriers. Captive companies also may give you greater input into decisions concerning defense strategies and settlements.

On the down side, some captive companies may not be as financially stable as their commercial counterparts. Because captive companies generally cover fewer policy holders, their distribution of risk is spread over a smaller population. This increases the risk of failure if the income from premiums is too low to cover expenses or if the company sustains losses that are higher than expected.

Beware of captive companies domiciled in offshore sites. Initially, many captive companies were formed in locations such as the Caribbean Islands to take advantage of tax breaks and relaxed regulations. Some of these companies, however, siphoned premiums out of the United States and subsequently disappeared, leaving many physicians with no coverage. Be sure you know who formed and operates a captive company before signing on.

Mutuals

A mutual insurance company is set up as a "cooperative" activity by a group of individuals who share in the profits and losses of the business. This type of insurance company has no stockholders or capital stock.

Risk-Retention Groups

Risk-retention groups are nonprofit, self-insuring corporations or associations formed for the sole purpose of providing insurance coverage to members or shareholders. Once licensed in a particular state, a risk-retention group may provide coverage to members in other states but has to abide only by the regulations of its home state. If you seek insurance coverage from a risk-retention group, be sure you know where it is licensed; such a group often is incorporated in a state with relatively lenient insurance regulations.

The premiums offered by risk-retention groups may be lower than those of other insurers. However, risk-retention groups are not covered by state guaranty funds, and, like insurance trusts, they may increase member premiums if losses are higher than expected.

Trusts

An insurance trust is a nonprofit legal entity that provides another way of spreading risk among policy holders. Medical liability trusts administer insurance programs on behalf of members. These companies may operate without the large cash reserve that is required of other carriers. For these reasons, trusts may have the advantage of lower premiums and operating costs.

Members of a trust place their personal assets on the line if claims exceed the funds available to pay them. This means that the trust may assess its members for additional payments—in addition to their premiums—if losses are higher than expected.

Because they are typically regulated through the state's department of corporations rather than the department of insurance, trusts are not protected by state guaranty funds. Trusts also generally have more stringent requirements for joining than do traditional companies because of the higher risk involved in operating without a large reserve.

Physician-Owned Companies

Physician-owned companies have proliferated in recent decades, insuring more than one half of U.S. physicians who buy their own insurance. These companies may be formed as trusts, captive companies, mutuals, risk-retention groups, or profit-making corporations. Many physician-owned companies are sponsored by state medical societies, and most are regulated under state insurance laws in the states where they were formed.

Physician-owned insurance companies tend to be sympathetic to and supportive of the professional problems of physicians, and they typically will defend a physician vigorously in the event of a lawsuit. This makes physician-owned carriers an appealing choice if you wish to have a greater say in claims decisions.

A disadvantage of physician-owned companies is that they generally provide coverage in only one state. However, some physician-owned companies are consolidating and are now licensed in several states.

Life Insurance

How much life insurance do you need? The answer varies according to your individual and family situation. The following three rules of thumb often are used as a guide for the amount of life insurance to buy:

1. Three to six times your annual income

2. An amount that, when invested, would yield earnings equal to 60–75% of your annual after-tax income

3. An amount that would pay off your own and your heirs' debts

As you get older, other guidelines for buying life insurance may come into play, such as to reduce your estate taxes.

Life insurance comes in two basic types: 1) term policies and 2) cash value policies. Death benefits paid to the beneficiary of either type of policy are not subject to federal income taxes.

TIP

Your insurance application is a part of the life insurance contract: an error on the application could result in no coverage at all.

Term Insurance

Term insurance is the least expensive type of life insurance and pays only a death benefit: if you die within the policy period, the death benefit set forth in the policy is paid to your designated beneficiary. The policy stays in force as long as you pay the premiums. If you do not renew the policy, there is no refund; the policy simply ends, and you are no longer insured.

The premiums for term insurance increase as you get older because the risk of your dying becomes greater. Some policies offer stable premiums for a period of years, ranging from 5 to 25 years. These policies may limit the renewal options. For example, a policy may offer stable premiums for 10 years but set an age limit for renewal, stating that it cannot be renewed if you have reached a certain age, such as 65 or 70 years. Check to see under what conditions the policy can be renewed at the end of the specified term.

Another type of term life insurance is called "level premium term" or "decreasing term." With this type, the premiums stay the same as you get older, but the death benefit decreases. Mortgage insurance is an example of decreasing term insurance: the premiums stay the same, but the amount of the benefit decreases each year as the mortgage principal decreases.

Cash-Value Insurance

Cash-value policies combine the payment of a death benefit with the accumulation of savings through an investment element. Most cash-value policies continue for indefinite periods as long as you pay the premiums.

Cash-value policies have higher premiums than those of term insurance because the investment component is an added value. Canceling your cash-value policy before 10–15 years results in significant financial penalties.

Listed as follows are the advantages of cash-value insurance:

- The cash value is tax-deferred

- You can borrow from the cash value of the policy

- You have the option of using the cash value to pay the premiums

- You can use the accumulated cash value to pay off the policy early

There are three types of cash-value insurance:

1. Whole life. The premiums of a whole-life policy usually are established according to your age at the time of enrollment, and the policy stays in effect until death as long as you continue to pay the premiums. The minimum cash value (face value) is guaranteed. Whole-life policies invest in relatively conservative instruments, such as U.S. Treasury bonds and certificates of deposit. The cash value accumulates at a predetermined rate during your lifetime. If you cancel (cash in) the policy, you receive the calculated cash value in a lump sum. You must pay income tax on the amount in excess of the premiums you paid. If you die, your beneficiary receives only the face value of the policy.

2. Universal life. This type of policy usually offers higher rates of return on investment than do whole-life policies. It also is more flexible than a whole-life policy: you can increase or decrease the death benefit (face value) by increasing or decreasing your premium, and you can use the cash value to pay the premiums.

3. Variable life. This kind of insurance usually has the same provisions as a universal life policy, but in addition you can choose the

investment vehicles of the policy. Variable-life policies let you invest in various types of funds, such as stocks, international funds, and bonds. However, the minimum cash value is not guaranteed. The potential returns are greater, but the risks also are greater.

Insurance Pitfalls To Avoid

Most experts advise against buying credit life insurance, such as mortgage insurance or a policy that will pay off a loan or credit balance if you die. The cost of these policies versus the benefit is not as great as simply increasing your life insurance to cover all of your current and anticipated debts when you die.

Do not buy more insurance than you need. Consider life insurance a way to manage risk, not an investment.

Do not switch insurance policies on the advice of an insurance agent. Agents work on commission and receive higher rates in the first year of a policy. The agent's commission is likely to be 50% of the first year's premium and 2–5% a year after that, so it is in the agent's interest to start you on a new policy. Change a cash-value policy only if the benefits outweigh the penalties for changing.

Disability Insurance

Disability insurance is very important, especially when you are young: your chance of becoming disabled at a young age is much higher than your chance of dying. A good disability policy will replace approximately 60–70% of your gross income.

As with all insurance products, however, shop for coverage that will meet your needs. If you have a source of income apart from your practice, you may be adequately covered with a disability policy that pays only a small amount each month.

TIP

If you have to choose between a higher monthly payment or a longer benefit period, choose the longer benefit period.

Definition of Disability

The single most important feature of a disability policy is the definition of disability. This definition determines when you are considered disabled so that you can begin receiving benefits under the policy.

The most favorable definition for you is one that defines disability as an inability to perform the duties of your occupation. This means the insurance will pay benefits if you cannot perform your duties as a practicing obstetrician–gynecologist. This type of coverage usually is more expensive.

Some policies define disability more narrowly, specifying that benefits would be paid only if you could not work in any occupation for which you are qualified or unable to work at all. Thus, if you could teach or consult with your disability, you would not receive benefits. Or, if you were able to see ambulatory patients but not do surgery or deliveries, for example, you would not receive benefits.

Exclusions

Some policies contain exclusions for certain causes of disability, such as suicide attempts, preexisting medical conditions, or disabilities incurred during a time of war. Check the exclusions carefully to be sure the insurance provides the protection you need. Some policies, for example, will not pay benefits if you have the human immunodeficiency virus (HIV) or if you become disabled as the result of pregnancy or childbirth.

Initiation and Term of Payments

When comparing provisions of disability policies, compare how long you must be disabled before benefits begin and how long the benefits last. Disability policies often let you chose the length of the waiting period before benefits start—typically a range from 30 to 180 days. The more quickly payments begin after you are disabled, the higher the premium. Choose coverage with the longest waiting period you can afford.

Most long-term disability policies run until age 65 years or death, whichever occurs first. Look for coverage for the longest benefit period that you can afford.

Coordination of Benefits

Some disability policies contain a clause regarding any disability benefits you might receive from Social Security or other disability insurance. Check to see if the policy pays the full disability benefit regardless of other benefits or if the amount is reduced by the amount of money you receive from other sources of disability payments. The premium will be higher for a policy that does not coordinate benefits.

Other Policy Provisions

Disability insurance products vary widely in the benefits they offer and the corresponding premiums. In considering disability insurance, look for the following provisions that may be included in the policy or may be offered as a rider—an option you can add for an increased premium:

- Receiving benefits, or partial benefits, if you are able to work part time

- Waiver of premiums while you are disabled

- Cost-of-living adjustment—an annual increase in benefits based on increases in the consumer price index

- Guarantee of renewability without a reevaluation of your health

- Catastrophic disability coverage—an increased level of benefits if you are cognitively impaired or require stand-by assistance

Group Policy Versus Individual Policy

If your group or employer provides disability coverage, you may still want to investigate purchasing your own disability policy. The terms of the group policy will likely be nonnegotiable and may include a definition of disability or a cap on the term of benefit payments that is not what you would like.

In addition, if your employer pays the premiums, any benefits you receive when you are dis-

abled will be taxed as income. If you pay your own premiums (and do not take the insurance premiums as a tax deduction), disability payment will not be taxed.

You may be able to negotiate a change in your compensation arrangement with your employer to forgo disability insurance as a fringe benefit, receiving instead the amount equal to the premium that the group would have paid. Be aware, however, that premiums for individual policies are much higher than those for group policies.

Disability Insurance for Overhead Expense

If you are in a solo practice, you also should consider overhead disability insurance, which is sometimes called business continuation insurance. This insurance will cover the costs of running your practice while you are disabled.

Policies offer a range of overhead coverage from which to choose. For example, the ACOG-endorsed insurance plan lets you choose a benefit of $1,000–$10,000 per month for up to 18 months while you are disabled.

You should choose coverage that matches your needs in case of disability. These include outlays for staff salaries, rent, utilities, and a locum tenens physician to fill in for you.

Health Insurance

You and your family need health insurance. Although many physicians offer professional courtesy discounts to other physicians and their families, many hospitals do not, and prescriptions can be costly.

The health care insurance industry, employer options, and government subsidies are all highly dynamic, so any list of available plans and their terms change rapidly. There are three major types of plans:

1. Traditional indemnity insurance. This type of health insurance uses fee-for-service reimbursement to cover hospitalization and medical or surgical services. The premiums for indemnity plans are the most expensive of

the major types of health insurance, but you are not limited to providers affiliated with the insurance plan. As the insured, you usually pay an annual deductible and a percentage, such as 20% or 25%, of the fees for services you receive. Prescription drugs in the plan's formulary also are covered, sometimes with a separate deductible.

2. Health maintenance organization (HMO). When you are enrolled in an HMO, medical and surgical services are paid as long as you receive care from a provider in the HMO. You usually have a co-payment of $5–20 for each visit. When you enroll, you select one primary care physician from the HMO's panel, and that provider must give you a written referral to a specialist in the HMO for your services from the specialist to be covered by the HMO.

3. Preferred provider organization. The premiums of a preferred provider organization plan usually are higher than those of an HMO. The trade-off is that you have more choice about the physicians you see, and you do not have to seek approval from your primary care physician first. Annual deductibles and co-payments also will vary.

Choose health plan features that match your needs. For example, you may want to enroll in an HMO, which is least expensive, if most of the physicians and the hospital you would go to participate in it. For example, if you or anyone in your family has a chronic illness or you plan to have a baby, consider how your premiums and out-of-pocket expenses for needed services and prescriptions would compare under each plan.

Annual deductibles are another feature to evaluate. You might want to increase your monthly cash flow by choosing a low-premium plan that has a high deductible.

Business Insurance

Business insurance is another type of insurance you should consider. If you are in solo practice, you will need several types of business insurance.

Property Insurance

Property insurance to cover your office and its contents in case of theft or fire is essential. If you are renting office space, check your lease to see if the landlord's insurance provides any coverage. Be sure the insurance covers the cost of restoring lost or damaged records.

Your property insurance will cover your computer equipment, but you may need a rider to cover loss of data or damage to the equipment as a result of power surges. If you use licensed software, talk to your software vendor about how much insurance you will need.

Liability Insurance

You should have liability coverage to protect your assets from lawsuits arising from accidents that occur on the premises of your office. Such liability usually is excluded from your medical liability insurance coverage. Commercial general liability coverage is a comprehensive type of insurance that covers you in case of lawsuits, including personal injury, product liability, advertising liability, and contractual liability.

Employee Dishonesty Insurance

Another type of coverage you should have as a practice owner is an employee fidelity bond, which protects you if an employee embezzles funds or steals equipment or supplies from your office. Such coverage is especially important when you are starting a practice, before you have procedures in place to minimize embezzlement opportunities (see Chapter 9 for details about creating such procedures).

An employee fidelity bond is inexpensive to buy. By purchasing a "blanket bond," you are covered for all office employees without having to specify names and update the policy every time staff members change.

Business Interruption Insurance

In addition to overhead insurance, you will need coverage if your office becomes inaccessible after a property loss, such as a fire, flood, or tornado.

Business interruption insurance pays you for lost revenue and ongoing expenses, such as rent or mortgage payments. Check to be sure that the policy covers expenses for a temporary office, moving, and notifying patients about the change in location.

Workers' Compensation

Workers' compensation insurance—coverage for the medical expenses and salary of any employee who is hurt or becomes ill on the job—is required in most states if you have three or more employees. Each state regulates benefits and costs, so most workers' compensation policies within your state will have identical coverage. Check that your policy is covered by your state's insurance insolvency fund.

Premiums are based on annual payroll estimates, including bonuses. Contact your state's Workers' Compensation Board for information about your responsibilities for providing this coverage. Your insurance agent or a consultant familiar with your state's workers' compensation rules also can help you purchase this insurance.

Umbrella Coverage

As a physician, it is a good idea for you to purchase umbrella insurance to protect your assets from judgments for personal liability that exceed normal coverage limits. Although you have liability insurance on your car, house, and office, you may want to talk to your agent about an umbrella policy, which can cover liability in excess of the stated amounts on those policies.

Sources of Information

Insurance Policies and Quotes

- The American College of Obstetricians and Gynecologists-endorsed insurance products offered through JLT Services Corporation: 800-214-8122

- American Medical Association wholly-owned subsidiary, AMA Insurance Agency, Inc: www.amainsure.com or 800-458-5736

- Insurance Information Institute: www.iii.org

- National Association of Insurance Commissioners provides links to each state insurance department's web site: www.naic.org/state_contacts/sid_websites.htm

- Physician Insurers Association of America, a trade association of more than 50 professional liability insurance companies owned and operated by physicians and dentists: www.piaa.us or (301) 947-9000

- Ryan Insurance Strategy Consultants (life and disability insurance): www.ryan-insurance.net or 800-796-0909

- Term life insurance: www.insweb.com, www.selectquote.com, or www.term4sale.com

Ratings of Insurance Companies

- A.M. Best Company: www.ambest.com or (908) 439-2200

- Moody's Investors Service: www.moodys.com

- Weiss Ratings: www.weissratings.com

Professional Liability Insurance

- American College of Obstetricians and Gynecologists' Professional Liability Department: 800-673-8444, ext 2582; e-mail liability@acog.org

- The Assistant: Information for Improved Risk Management, published by ACOG: sales.acog.org or 800-762-2264

- Litigation Assistant: A Guide for the Defendant Physician, 2nd ed., published by ACOG: sales.acog.org or 800-762-2264

- Professional Liability and Risk Management: An Essential Guide for Obstetricians and Gynecologists, published by ACOG: sales.acog.org or 800-762-2264

Chapter 7. Personal Skills

Negotiating

Negotiating skills are useful in many areas. You need such skills in negotiating contracts, of course, but they also can help you resolve situations with patients, your spouse or significant other, your colleagues, lenders, and managed care organizations.

In some situations, often referred to as a zero sum game, when one party gains, the other party loses. If you do not expect to deal with individuals again and you do not need their goodwill, using an aggressive negotiating style—seeking to win while the other individual loses—might be appropriate.

In many important negotiations, you are negotiating a relationship, not a transaction. In these cases, effective negotiators are collaborative. For example, when you are negotiating an employment contract to join a group practice, you are not just trying to get the best deal for yourself; you also want the best deal for the group, which will soon be your group.

Reaching a "win-win" agreement is an appropriate goal for maintaining a good working relationship after the negotiation is concluded. In a win-win agreement, both parties feel positive about the outcome.

Preparation

Do your homework before approaching a negotiation. Assess your own goals and take time to find out as much as you can about the other party and the issues involved:

> *In many important negotiations, you are negotiating a relationship, not a transaction.*

- Research the other party. Find out all you can about the other party. If you will be negotiating with a group practice, read everything on its web site and ask to have any marketing literature or patient handouts about the practice sent to you in advance. Check to see if any of the physicians have published articles or reports.

- Investigate alternatives. Plan to go into negotiations knowing what alternatives you have. Your best alternative to a negotiated agreement is the option you will take if the negotiation fails.

If you are negotiating an employment contract, for instance, this may be an offer from another practice or it could be to stay where you are. Determining your best alternative to a negotiated agreement beforehand protects you from accepting a poor offer and puts you in a stronger negotiating position.

- Unbundle the issues. Break the agreement to be negotiated into small parts. In dealing with an employment contract, for instance, break compensation down into its smallest components, such as salary, moving costs, bonuses, and reimbursed expenses.

- Anticipate the other party's wants and needs. Try to determine what the top issues are for the other party. This will help you develop strategies to negotiate your position. Estimate the other party's probable limits in reaching a compromise. Consider your counterpart's best alternative to a negotiated agreement—what is likely to be his or her next best choice?

- Establish your bargaining range. Identify objectives for each of the issues you have unbundled by setting an optimum, minimum, and target goal. The minimum is the point at which you would walk away from the offer if the other party cannot meet your request. The optimum is your starting point—the best deal, one you see as ideal but something that is not outrageous. The target is the point where you would like to end up after negotiations.

- Identify your leveraging points. Determine the areas most important to you. Use those that you do not care much about as leverage in negotiating to achieve your priorities. Also, identify the attributes you bring to the table. For example, in joining a practice, you may have special training the practice needs or be fluent in a language spoken by a large percentage of its patients.

- Identify the decision maker. If you will be negotiating with several individuals, identify the individual who is the authorized decision maker. Do not get into a situation in which someone can say, in effect, that he or she has to "check with the boss on that." You want to talk directly with the individual who has the authority to make agreements.

TIPS

Write down your negotiating limits beforehand, and stick to them.

Save the most important items you want to negotiate for the end.

Negotiating Strategies

The following techniques may be useful when you negotiate:

- Convey confidence. You have done your homework. You know your own goals and your best alternative to a negotiated agreement. Throughout the negotiation process, remind yourself of your own objectives to help you stay focused. To a great extent, power is a matter of perception. Do not act cocky but avoid being obsequious or overly appreciative that the other party has agreed to negotiate with you. You may feel at a disadvantage when negotiating with a more powerful individual, but keep in mind that you would not be negotiating unless you have something the other party needs.

- Set the stage for agreement. Establish rapport with the other party early in the negotiation by looking for areas on which you both agree. Bring up points on which you are fairly certain the other party can say "yes." Agreement helps establish a foundation of trust and respect that will be useful when you address more controversial topics.

- Ask open-ended questions. Try to avoid questions that can be answered with a "yes" or "no." Your goal in the early stages of negotiation is to find out more about what the other party's real needs are. If you are negotiating an employment contract, you have been offered the position, but you may not know what you have that is most desired or important to the practice. Bring to bear all that you learned earlier in the interviewing process.

- Listen. Be wary of talking too much. By listening more than you talk, you will uncover information and attitudes that can help you understand the other party's concerns and interests.

- Restate comments. Paraphrase the other party's statements in your own words. This lets the other party provide clarification or correct misinterpretations. Often you will hear an elaboration on a point that will help you uncover negotiable areas.

- Depersonalize disagreements. When identifying points to be negotiated, refer to them objectively rather than assigning ownership to the other party. For instance, instead of saying "the way you assign call hours," say "the structure of call coverage." Otherwise, the other party is likely to feel defensive.

- Separate defining problems from exploring solutions. Seek to clarify an issue and evaluate the nature of the disagreement before exploring solutions. Discussing solutions before the issues are fully defined can lead to confusion and to restating problems and renegotiating agreements made prematurely.

- Do not legitimize a bad offer. If the other party's initial offer is outrageous or truly unacceptable, do not make a counteroffer. Doing so could help establish an unacceptable range for negotiation. Try broadening the discussion instead by probing the other party's position and working to refocus the overall goal of the negotiation.

- Do not compare offers. Although you have researched alternatives and know what someone else might be offering you, discuss the current deal on its merits. Do not compare it openly with other offers you have. Other offers you may have are your backup if you cannot reach a satisfactory agreement in the current negotiations.

- Do not issue an ultimatum. Any kind of "take it or leave it" or "this is my final position" pronouncement cuts off the negotiations completely. Ultimatums are especially dangerous early in the negotiating process.

- Use deferment as a trade-off. In negotiating an employment contract, compensation is an area in which you can sometimes gain what you want by deferring it to the second year. For example, if your goal is a first-year salary of $120,000, but the practice is firm on offering only $110,000, suggest that the $10,000 difference be added to your second-year's salary. Making this suggestion gives you the opportunity to make it clear that you are thinking long-term and conveys your confidence that the practice will be happy with you. Thus, if the second-year salary was to be $130,000, indicate you will accept the $110,000 offered for the first year if they make the salary $140,000 in year 2.

- Use your leverage. Do not let any of the leveraging points you identified go unexpressed during negotiations. In the preparation stage, you identified the attributes you have that they want. Now is the time to bring them up.

- Bring material that supports your position. Data and literature convey authority. Bring reports that back up your negotiating points, such as salary surveys. If you want to work part time, for example, bring articles that discuss the success stories and the benefits that such arrangements can offer.

- Beware of a stall—reach closure. If the other party seems to be uninterested in finalizing the agreement, it could mean he or she thinks delaying the deal might improve his or her bargaining position. Ask what additional information is needed for a final decision to be made.

Evaluate Yourself

Negotiating situations will continue throughout your life. Learn from them. After any negotiating process, evaluate your performance. Ask yourself the following questions:

- What additional preparation could I have done?

- Did I communicate clearly?

- Were options explored sufficiently?

- Did the outcome meet each party's real needs?

Team Building

In health care, most work is done by teams. Having the skills to work within a team and to lead a team is important.

Creating a Team Culture

Teams often represent different work groups, and individuals have different training, perspectives, and work cultures. Examples include a hospital quality improvement team that is assembled from various departments and an office practice made up of clinical and administrative staff or physicians and clerical personnel.

The challenge in building an effective team is to develop a team culture in which everyone works toward a common goal. In an office practice, for example, a team might be assembled with the goal to decrease patient waiting times, reduce paperwork, or develop an adolescent health care program.

Everyone on the team can and should be empowered to work toward the goal in his or her own job, in addition to contributing ideas for the team as a whole. Physicians often try to have all the answers—your instinct and training have geared you to solve problems—but the individual doing a particular job is the best individual to fix problems and offer new ideas about it.

If you are the leader of the team, make sure the following attributes are in place:

- All the team members know the goal.

- Everyone has ways to communicate with each other.

- Team members understand their own role and the roles of others.

- Individual skills of team members are valued by others.

- Members have resources available to accomplish their tasks.

- There are mechanisms in place to measure results.

Important elements for building an effective team are establishing trust and shared accountability. Team members need to trust the other team members, feel ownership in the outcome the team is working toward, and have a sense of responsibility to the team. Effectively building a team or contributing to a team also requires using effective communication skills. These elements of a team culture can take time to establish.

Leading and Managing Teams

Management theorists point out that leading and managing are two different dynamics. Leadership involves having a vision and influencing others to work toward it; a leader makes people want to achieve. Management is the process of ensuring that tasks are accomplished. Team building requires both leadership and management skills.

The team leader has the responsibility to provide the following elements for creating effective teams:

- Goals and expectations. The team leader must provide clarity and structure. Tell your team what you expect of them but also invite them to set goals for themselves and contribute ideas for the team project. Individuals do better when they perceive goals to be their own. Some expectations may relate to their regular job duties; others may be one-time assignments specific to the team goal. Challenging and specific goals result in more effort than do easy or vague goals.

- Motivation. You motivate someone to work toward goals by giving them the rewards they want. Discovering the personal goals and expectations of individual team members can help you motivate them. The key is to arrange for individuals to achieve their own goals while working toward the group goals.

- Empowerment. Trust individuals with important tasks. Invite team members to indicate areas in which they would like to take initiative. Empower them by giving them the freedom to exercise their own discretion. This requires accepting others for who they are, being creative, and accepting risk. Individuals who feel empowered have greater job satisfaction, generate more ideas, and perform better.

- Resources. Discuss what is required to get the job done and be sure the resources are available. Consider individuals, education, equipment, research, and other resources needed to reach the goal.

- Education. A team goal may involve education, such as training on a new computer system, learning Health Insurance Portability and Accountability Act requirements, or studying conversational Spanish. Taking classes or going to a seminar together can foster a sense of team spirit.

- Cross-training. Working together on a project presents a great opportunity for individuals to expand their understanding of what other individuals do in their jobs. Foster a culture of constant learning among your team, including learning about each other's regular responsibilities.

- Feedback. Providing feedback on performance is a basic tenet of motivation. A monthly report related to the overall goal is one way to do this (eg, a report of the number of medical records converted to a new system or the average patient waiting times).

- Positive reinforcement. Champion your team members. Encourage them when they are down. Praise them when they do well. Thank them for their contributions both individually and to the team as a whole.

Effective and Productive Meetings

Meetings provide an opportunity to cement team norms and facilitate positive relationships and communication. Although information sharing can and should take place outside meetings, regular meetings offer opportunities for problem solving, reporting on progress, and building a sense of team spirit and cohesion.

A good meeting is one in which team goals are introduced or reinforced and solutions are generated. A meeting needs a facilitator to guide but not direct individuals' participation. The following factors can contribute to effective meetings:

- Use an agenda. Make an agenda with the anticipated times for each topic. Everyone should know what the agenda is. If it is a short meeting or quickly planned and there is no time to make copies and distribute them beforehand, put the agenda on a flipchart or board that you and others can refer to during the meeting. At the end of each meeting, invite individuals to name topics for the next meeting and invite them to contact you before the next meeting if they have topics for the group.

- Give adequate notice. Allow time for participants to receive the notice and prepare. If the agenda is not finalized, give advance notice of the time and place and indicate that the agenda will follow.

- Do not meet just because it is scheduled. If there are no issues to discuss, do not hold the meeting just because it is Tuesday and that is when you always meet.

- Limit the meeting time. Use the timed agenda to stay on track. If the discussion goes off on a tangent, repeat the objectives of the meeting or the topic at hand. If it becomes clear that a topic needs more time, put the issue on the next scheduled meeting, or if appropriate, schedule a separate meeting to address it.

- Structure input. Meetings can be a way to foster teamwork and participation. Make different individuals responsible for different agenda items. If discussion reveals that more information is needed, assign tasks and have the responsible individuals report at the next meeting.

- Facilitate discussion. Work diligently to be sure everyone's ideas are heard and that no one dominates the discussion. If two individuals seem to talk only to each other and not the group on a certain item, invite others to comment; if the issue involves only the two individuals, suggest that they continue to work on that topic outside the meeting and report back.

- Set ground rules. Keep meetings constructive; they should not be gripe sessions. Do not issue reprimands and make it clear that the meeting is to be positive and is intended for updates, analysis, problem solving, and decision making. Create an environment in which disagreement and alternative perspectives are acceptable. When individuals do offer opposing opinions, facilitate open discussion that focuses on issues and not personalities.

- Circulate a meeting summary before the next meeting. Formal minutes are appropriate for some meetings. At the very least, a brief summary of actions should be prepared, including decisions reached and assignments made, with deadlines.

Conflict Management and Resolution

Conflict is not the same as disagreement. Disagreement within a team is healthy, and individuals should be encouraged to express differing opinions in open discussion of a topic. Conflict should not be suppressed or ignored.

Conflicts have many underlying causes, including personality differences, resentment arising from a perception of inequity, or a perceived or real threat to an individual's self-esteem or power. Conflict does not always manifest itself in outward actions. Thus, conflict occurs when a comment by someone else makes you angry, whether or not you express that anger or the other individual is even aware of it.

Managing Yourself in Conflicts

Managing conflict requires you to be aware of your own reactions, realize that you have choices about how to react, and control your choice rather than reacting automatically. When you exercise such choice, you are taking responsibility—you are empowering yourself. If you do otherwise, you surrender choice and disempower yourself. You should consider the following approach to examining your reactions to conflict:

- Identify your feelings. Although it is difficult, the most important first step in managing conflict is to focus on what is going on inside you instead of focusing on the other individual. Practice paying attention to what you are thinking and feeling. What is the unspoken message you are inferring from a situation, such as "they do not like me," or "she thinks I am a bad doctor." Identifying how you are interpreting someone's behavior will help you understand what your hot buttons are that someone else can push to evoke a response.

- Do not lash out. When we feel anger or resentment, it is natural to lash out and blame the other individual, but this simply escalates the conflict.

- Express your feelings. Others often are unaware of or underestimate how hurt or angry you are about a situation. Express as clearly as you can to the other party how you feel or how a situation has affected you. Be sure the language you use is not inflammatory or rude. Suppress the desire to punish or blame. Rather than saying what the other individual should or should not do, express your own feelings or perspective using statements beginning with "I." Your goal is to convey what you need, not to force the other individual to fix things. Assertively expressing your needs and feelings is not the resolution to the conflict; it is the beginning. The other individual may, in fact, react defensively, even though you have stated only your perspective and not accused or found fault. Your goal at first should be to help the other individual see you as an individual with feelings and needs that are affected by the other's behavior or by the situation.

- Consider the other. You also must honestly assess whether you are open to broader views. It takes courage to do this, but you cannot expect it of others if you do not do it yourself. Remind yourself that each individual's perspective must be given consideration and respect to reach a solution. Find out what matters to the other party. Ask thoughtful questions about what he or she wants and feels to be important.

Responding to Criticism

A specific type of conflict is complaints or criticism from others. Criticism may come from patients, other obstetrician–gynecologists, consultants, nurses, or hospital administrators.

Be alert to signs of anger or frustration—a raised voice, clenched fists, vehement language, crying, or being on the verge of crying. If someone criticizes you emotionally, deal with the emotion first. Individuals raise their voices because they think they are not being heard, in the sense of being understood. Do not start justifying or defending your behavior. Your defense or denial will serve only to inflame individuals more.

Acknowledge their emotion, telling them that you are hearing or seeing how angry or upset they are. Accurately label the emotions as you perceive them. Make statements such as "I can see how upset you are," "You feel like you cannot deal with it," or "So you are really angry when this happens." Stay in this active listening and empathizing mode until the individual has calmed down.

Once the heat is out of the interchange, draw the individual out to learn all you can about what is behind the emotion. Acknowledge the individual's perceptions. This does not mean you agree

but that you register his or her perspective. In resolving criticism directed at you, be sure you know what is the actual complaint.

Finally, ask what the individual would really like to happen and explore options for remedies. Find out what could be done now to make it okay again.

Mediating Conflict

Because situations involving conflict are common in health care, you may be called on to settle a dispute. Patient complaints are increasingly being brought to mediation with the use of an uninvolved physician, or you may be aware of a conflict between office staff members and be in a position to mediate. Avoid the temptation to take responsibility for resolving the conflict; as a mediator, your role is to help the parties in conflict explore acceptable options and develop agreement using the following techniques:

- Establish a win-win approach to resolution. Define your mediator role as one of supporting "winning" for both parties. As in negotiating, a key to success is for the parties to change from thinking of the other as an adversary to considering him or her a partner in reaching a solution. When both individuals win, both are committed to the solution because it actually suits them.

- Create a constructive foundation. Use caring language. Create an environment in which individuals feel safe to open up. Actively discourage judgments about who is right and who is wrong. If necessary, set ground rules that prohibit behavior such as put-downs, blaming, threats, bringing up the past, or getting even.

- Define the issue in neutral terms. Take personalities out of the problem definition. For example, state the problem as "filing" rather than "whether Erin or Wendy should handle filing." Be prepared to revise the statement of the issue as your understanding of the conflict evolves. Resist advising. Your role is to steer the process, not the content.

Be objective even when only one party is present.

- Identify underlying needs. Invite both parties to state their impression of the problem at hand. Find out what matters to them. Ask thoughtful questions about what they want and what is important to them. Focus on the "why," not the "what." An individual's position usually is based on a deeper interest or need, so listen carefully to explore the hidden or underlying assumptions of each party. The better you understand why something matters to individuals, the better you will be able to explore options that will satisfy their real interests.

- Probe feelings. If they do not express their feelings, solicit the information: "How did that affect you?" or "How did you feel about that?" Assess nonverbal cues as well as what is said.

- Collect information. In addition to finding out about the individuals' needs and concerns, obtain background information. Be sure the facts are all out in the open. Ask questions about details that have not been expressed: "How much does it cost? What happens when…? How often does this happen?" If someone says, "I do not like it," ask for details about what aspects he or she objects to.

- Check understanding. Paraphrase what you hear the parties saying, and at various points, ask each to state what he or she heard the other individual say. Sometimes individuals are surprised when they hear their perspective articulated by someone else.

- Engage them in problem solving. Invite the parties to suggest ways to reach agreement. Ask them to list their choices and the consequences of each.

- Add objectivity. Focus on the issue, not on personalities. Reinterpret an attack on an individual to focus it on the issue. This will help individuals not to be defensive. Where possible, turn to outside sources for guidance. Published guidelines, whether for salaries, job duties, or clinical practice, can bring objectivity to bear and help take the discussion out of the realm of emotion. Using objective resources also may make it possible for an individual to back down without feeling humiliated by justifying a change in position because of new information.

- Reach consensus. Identify the solutions that seem to have the greatest potential to address the interests of all parties. Lay out the solutions for discussion, watching for cues from all parties about which options are most appealing. The parties must believe the agreement is fair and recognize that they have gained something.

Communication

Effective communication requires paying attention to an entire process, not just the message you want to convey, whether through writing or speaking. To communicate effectively, you have to overcome potential barriers that exist in each of the following components of the communication process:

- Sender. Be aware of how your own attitudes, emotions, knowledge, and credibility with the receiver might impede or alter whether and how your message is received.

- Medium. Choose the right medium for the message (eg, e-mail, telephone call, personal visit, notes in the margin, or a typed review). Sometimes more than one medium is appropriate, such as when you give the patient written material to reinforce what you have said or when you follow-up a telephone call with an e-mail.

- Setting. For oral communication, the setting can be critical to communicating effectively. Is a chat in the corridor okay or should this be a closed-door discussion? Should you meet in your office or over lunch?

- Message. Make sure what you communicate, whether oral or written, is organized, is not too complex for the medium and the receiver, and does not contain errors. One of the biggest pitfalls is offering too much information too fast.

- Receiver. Consider the knowledge and biases of the individual with whom you are communicating.

When you communicate in person, be aware of your own and the listener's body language, such as eye contact, facial expressions, posture, and gestures. Your tone of voice, loudness, and pitch communicate a message than can be much stronger than the words used. Pay attention to personal space—do not invade an individual's personal space by getting too close.

Writing

Whether you are sending an e-mail message, writing a letter in response to a patient complaint, or preparing an article for publication, the most important aspect of writing is the reader. What biases does your reader have? Where will the reader be when he or she receives your writing? How important is your message to the reader?

The purpose of writing is to change the reader. You want the reader to do something, to know something, or to feel something so write in a way that helps the reader as well as yourself (Box 7–1).

Be Clear

Say what you mean and mean what you say. Very often when writing is not clear it is because you are trying to avoid saying something (Box 7–2).

BOX 7-1 BENEFITS OF EFFECTIVE WRITING

- Forces you to examine your views
- Reinforces qualities needed in medicine: logic, clarity, accuracy
- Helps others understand your intended message
- Reflects positively on you

BOX 7-2 REASONS FOR INEFFECTIVE WRITING

- Did not consider the reader sufficiently
- Disorganization
- Tried to avoid saying something
- Tried to impress rather than inform
- Was careless (did not sufficiently edit, revise, reorganize, proofread)

Writers must constantly ask, "What am I trying to say and have I said it?"

Go back through what you have written to see if there is anything that could be misinterpreted. Does it raise unanswered questions or fail to make your point?

Use organization to help you communicate your message. Put your main point first. It is a common pitfall to lay out the background information as an introduction and wait until the end to make your conclusion. Here is where thinking about your reader can help you. Will your reader stick with you until the final paragraph, or maybe page two, to find out your point? If extensive background information is needed, separate it and make it an attachment that you refer to. This makes the main body of your text more concise.

Use the appearance and format to help the reader grasp your message. Long, dense paragraphs are a turn-off. For any sentence that enumerates items, convert the items to a list with bullets. Use subheads for different sections in any written piece longer than a page.

Be Concise

Effective writing is concise. It does not waste the reader's time.

- Delete redundant words. Scrutinize your writing to be sure you have not fallen into the trap of using redundant expressions, such as past history, close proximity, proposed plan, or important essential.

- Cut out wordy phrases. Avoid using clunky and dead phrases when one word will do (Box 7–3).

BOX 7–3 BE CONCISE INSTEAD OF WORDY

Wordy	*Concise*
at the present time	now
in the event that	if
referred to as	called
with the exception of	except
for the reason that	because
for the purpose of	for
in order to	to
on a daily basis	daily
the month of December	December
relative to	about
in regard to	about
based on the fact that	because
during the course of	during

- Watch for deadwood sentence introductions. Do not begin sentences with phrases that can be dropped without losing any meaning, such as "It should be pointed out that…," "It is significant that…," "It is essential that…," "It is evident that…," and "It should be remembered that…"

- Avoid bloated, jargony, or pretentious language. Do not turn off your reader with clichés, journalese, legalese, corporatese, or medicalese. Your writing should sound natural, like you talk. Granted, writing usually is not as colloquial as oral communication, which often includes sentence fragments or slang that are not acceptable in written communication. But just as you would not say "Enclosed in the refrigerator please find the leftover meatloaf," do not write "Enclosed please find the map for the party." Instead, write "The map is enclosed," or "I have attached the map."

- Avoid passive voice. Sentences using the active voice are 20–30% shorter than those with the passive voice. In addition, use of the passive voice is less clear and leads to awkward constructions and misunderstandings. The active voice conveys more energy than the passive voice. Say "The residents presented the awards," not "The awards were presented by the residents."

Be Correct

Your reader will judge you by your writing and in some cases judge your practice or others whom you represent. Fair or not, the reader uses your writing to decide how credible you are, how smart you are, and how careful you are. Be correct in your writing not only by having your facts right, but also by using correct grammar, spelling, word choice, and punctuation. Once something is in written form, it cannot be taken back.

Always take time to go back through what you have written. Whether it is a grant proposal, a letter of recommendation, a meeting summary, or a congratulatory e-mail message, check that your facts are accurate, no extra words were left in as you edited, your pronouns have antecedents, and names are spelled correctly.

Common errors in writing are in number agreement, parallel construction, misplaced modifiers, punctuation, and spelling. Malapropisms can set you up for ridicule. "The survey results are skewered" or "There is a true medical liability crisis brooding" can be amusing to the reader but nevertheless reflect on your writing abilities. Read over your writing to be sure it is correct. Never allow something you have dictated to be mailed or published without your review.

Using the wrong word is an especially common error. We often do not know the exact meaning of the words we use or are not aware of the "evil twins" that can render our prose incorrect. A few examples of the hundreds of words often used incorrectly include affect/effect, allude/refer, imminent/eminent, assure/ensure, born/borne, and discreet/discrete.

Virtually all style guides contain extensive glossaries of such troublesome expressions, explain their distinctions, and give examples of correct use. Online help also is available by searching for the term "word usage."

E-mail

E-mail has numerous features that make it a wonderful tool for communicating. It is immediate; it is automatically time-stamped; and filing and organizing are easy.

The e-mail subject line is an especially useful feature that is typically underused. Make it your best friend. Use it like a newspaper headline to draw the reader in and convey your main point or alert the reader to a deadline. For example, instead of using "PROM" in the subject, the more helpful subject line "Plan to discuss PROM this Friday—see article attached" alerts the reader to be prepared to discuss the topic at an upcoming meeting.

Put the most important information—the purpose of the e-mail—in the first paragraph. Also, do not forget to supply appropriate contact information, including telephone numbers or alternative e-mail addresses, for responses or questions.

Except among friends who know you well, stay away from sarcasm in e-mail messages. Also, in most cases it is better to offer criticism in person or in a telephone call than to do so in e-mail. In an e-mail message, the receiver does not have the benefit of your tone of voice and body language to help interpret your communication and consequently supplies the missing tone and attitude. Thus, something you wrote with good intentions and an open mind or even with humor can be interpreted as nitpicky, negative, and destructive.

Because we use e-mail for its speed, it is easy to get in the habit of dashing off a message and hitting the "send" button. We count on the automatic spell-check (and you should have it turned on as your default option) to catch your typos. But spelling errors are the least of the problems in communicating effectively. Go back to the basic rule of effective writing: concern for the reader. Read through your message. Is it clear? Is it organized? Is it concise? The very speed with which we dash off e-mail messages makes e-mail the place in which we are most likely to communicate poorly.

Listening

Effective listening does not just happen. It takes work. If you do not cultivate good listening skills, the result often is misconception and misunderstanding. Moreover, the speaker is likely to feel dismissed.

Ineffective listening habits are especially troublesome in medical practice. Communication issues are at the crux of many medical malpractice claims. Liability aside, every patient needs to know you are listening to her. Some of the biggest pitfalls that can interfere with effective physician–patient communication are feigning attention, allowing distractions, and dismissing what she is saying as unimportant.

Listed as follows are ways to improve your listening skills:

- Look at the speaker; pay attention to nonverbal cues.
- Do not interrupt; let the speaker finish.
- Give your full attention to the speaker; with patients, do not page through the medical record while she is speaking. In other settings, avoid looking at what else is going on in the room.
- Focus on content, not delivery.
- Listen for main points, often mentioned at the beginning or end.
- Give feedback—nod now and then to show that you understand.
- If appropriate, take notes—do not trust your memory.
- Empathize—try to see the speaker's point of view. Affirm that you have heard her perspective or that you understand her feelings.
- Repeat in your own words what the speaker said.
- Invite elaboration and ask for clarification.

Time Management

Managing your time effectively has two main elements: 1) mission and 2) efficiency. There is no point in gaining efficiency to accomplish more if what you are accomplishing does not move you toward your goal. If you are not doing the "right" things, it does not matter how much you get done.

Set Goals

Make a list of what you value—what is important to you. Then, keep an activity log for several days, writing down everything you do in very small blocks of time, such as every 15 minutes. After you have logged your time for a few days, analyze the length of time you spend on various activites. Ask yourself if what you did reflects what you believe is important. Although your daily routine cannot always reflect your priorities, this exercise may help you reflect on what is important. You have a variety of roles and priorities. Assess how well your roles are balanced to meet your goals.

Take time to define your goals, both short term and long term. Short-term goals are ones you aim for in the next year. Five years is probably a good range for your long-term goals. You may want to set goals for several categories of life, such as family, physical fitness, and pleasure. However, you will lose focus if you set too many goals. Choose one, two, or three goals as priorities. Write down your goals and add some specificity, such as an achievement you want to reach by a certain date. Make your goals realistic.

Once you decide what matters to you the most, work on the skills and discipline to pursue your goals. Goals usually are intangible. Convert such goals into small actions, and schedule them. Whether your goal is to write a novel, spend more time with your family, develop a new surgery skill, or become more physically fit, you need to set concrete, achievable objectives to work toward it, so that "writing a novel" becomes "write every day from 7:30 to 8:30" or "register for the 8-week creative writing workshop at the community college." The goal of increasing time with family becomes "pick Rachel up from school at 3:30 on Thursdays and spend one-on-one time doing something she chooses." Schedule the concrete objectives on your calendar, right along with your business meetings and surgery schedule.

Find Balance

Physicians traditionally are very work centered, sometimes sacrificing time for family and personal emotional needs. Medicine and many other professions have a culture of glorifying long hours and high productivity.

Although that work-versus-personal-life model seems to be changing, it is still very easy, especially in the early years of trying to establish yourself in practice, to focus excessively on work at the expense of play, personal development, or other goals. Moreover, the ethic of medicine is caring for patients, and you are in medicine because you do care and receive personal satisfaction from that. You take pride in giving of yourself to your patients, so it can be doubly hard to limit the energy you devote to patient care and building your practice. Without a balance between your personal development and your work, however, you are likely to experience burnout, which can lead to resentment of patients as well as personally destructive behavior, estrangement from loved ones, and illness.

If you are just finishing residency training, moving to a new location, changing practices, or changing careers, it is an ideal time to take stock of your life, contemplate your values, and enumerate your goals. You may feel your life has been (or still is) "on hold" while you finish residency or continue to work in a location or a practice that you are planning to leave. Do not fall into the trap of thinking that the forthcoming change will, in and of itself, fix things or bring the personal enrichment into your life that has been in abeyance.

Be Efficient

Like most individuals, you probably respond to a sense of urgency, which typically is imposed by others. The "outside world"—telephone calls, meetings, mail—thrusts itself on you, and it is tempting to respond to whatever is at hand. If you do not set your own priorities and goals and develop a plan to achieve them, you will continue to simply do what is expected of you by others. In addition, personal habits—overcommitment, procrastination, lack of planning—can add to the sense that you are too busy to accomplish what is really important to you.

Listed as follows are tips for improving your efficiency in practice:

- Prune your calendar. Drop memberships, committees, and meetings that do not provide real benefit to you or your practice.

- Delegate. Many tasks—both clinical and administrative—can be delegated. Train someone else to take the patient history. Tasks such as opening mail waste your time. Where possible, assign meeting attendance and handling correspondence to the office manager.

- Develop standard information for patients. Use handouts and brochures for patient education and standard discharge instruction sheets. Written information not only saves time in responding to inquiries later, but it helps the patient.

- Process paperwork efficiently. Use preprinted forms for histories, physicals, and progress notes. Do not write out notes that can be handled by check boxes. Use preprinted prescription forms for your 20 most commonly prescribed medications. Schedule time each day for administrative tasks; if you do not do it every day you will fall behind. Also, your delays can drive up the costs of support staff because they become less efficient by having to remind you, respond to inquiries from others, or delay doing their part of a job until they hear back from you. Try to process every piece of paper on your desk within 24 hours. If possible, handle each item just once—do not look at it and set it aside to deal with later.

- Use to-do lists and prioritize. Buy a task organizer or just keep a simple to-do list. Prioritize the list, so you are ready to do what is next on the list if you have a no-show, for example. Otherwise, it is too easy to go back to your office and waste time while you decide what to do next. Break down large projects into their components. There is no single way that makes a to-do list most efficient. Make it work for you, whether that means writing tasks for each day in your calendar, creating a list for the week, keeping it on your computer, using colored highlights, or whatever.

- Batch your work. Set aside specific times for similar tasks, such as reading mail and returning telephone calls. It is more efficient to make five phone calls consecutively than to make them separately. Work on one project at a time.

- Group similar patient visits. You can work more quickly if you do all of the same kind of patient visits consecutively (eg, bundle your prenatal appointments for the same day or the same morning).

- Learn speed reading. Take a speed-reading course—most are just a couple hours and will help you save many hours of time. One of the first things you will learn is what not to read.

- Use your voice mail for reminders. If you need to bring something to the office from home or vice-versa, record a message to yourself about it.

Sources of Information

- The American Management Association offers books, courses, and self-study programs on all topics covered in this chapter: www.amanet.org

Negotiating

- *The Negotiator Magazine,* a free on-line magazine: www.negotiatormagazine.com

- *Bargaining for Advantage: Negotiation Strategies for Reasonable People*, by G. Richard Shell

- *Getting to Yes: Negotiating Agreement Without Giving In*, by Roger Fisher, William Ury, and Bruce Patton

Team Building

- *A Passion for Excellence: The Leadership Difference*, by Tom Peters
- *The Leadership Challenge: How to Keep Getting Extraordinary Things Done in Organizations*, by James M. Kouzes, Barry Z. Posner, and Tom Peters
- *The Wisdom of Teams: Creating the High Performance Organization*, by Jon R. Katzenbach and Douglas K. Smith
- *Intrinsic Motivation at Work: Building Energy and Commitment*, by Kenneth W. Thomas
- *1001 Ways to Reward Employees*, by Bob Nelson
- *Meetings: Do's, Don'ts, and Donuts*, by Sharon Lippincott

Conflict Management

- *The Eight Essential Steps to Conflict Resolution: Preserving Relationships at Work, at Home, and in the Community*, by Dudley Weeks
- *Managing Differences*, by Daniel Dana
- *When Generations Collide*, by Lynne C. Lancaster and David Stillman

Communication

- *The Elements of Style*, 4th ed, by William Strunk, Jr, E.B. White, and Roger Angell
- *The Chicago Manual of Style: The Essential Guide for Writers, Editors, and Publishers*, 15th ed, by University of Chicago Press staff
- *American Medical Association Manual of Style*, 9th ed., published by the American Medical Association
- *On Writing Well, 25th Anniversary: The Classic Guide to Writing Nonfiction*, by William Zinsser
- *Genderspeak: Men, Women, and the Gentle Art of Verbal Self-Defense*, by Suzette Haden Elgin
- *Time to Think: Listening to Ignite the Human Mind*, by Nancy Kline
- *Listen Up: Hear What's Really Being Said*, by Jim Dugger

Time Management

- *The Complete Idiot's Guide to Managing Your Time*, by Jeff Davidson
- *First Things First*, by Stephen Covey and Rebecca Merrill
- *Make Success Measurable: A Mindbook-Workbook for Setting Goals and Taking Action*, by Douglas K. Smith

Chapter 8.   Practice Operations

The Physician's Role

The physician has to strike a balance between the extremes of micro-managing tasks and delegating all management responsibilities to an office manager. As the owner or one of the owners of a practice, your responsibilities are like those of a corporate board:

- Set policy and standards

- Hire staff to implement policy and perform needed tasks

- Ensure reporting mechanisms are in place for you to monitor performance of the practice

See Box 8–1 for a checklist of a healthy practice.

If you are joining an established practice, you may have little input at first into the office policies and hiring decisions. However, you are viewed as an authority figure by staff and patients and should have a clear understanding of practice operations. Familiarize yourself with the procedure and employee manuals and review each employee's position description to help understand individual responsibilities and how the functions interrelate. You also should have an understanding of laws and statutes regulating medical practice (see Chapter 10 for more information).

Personnel Issues

People are the most important asset of a medical practice and represent the largest single expense in a practice. Getting the right individuals for the right positions is essential for an efficient and successful practice.

Employee Manual

Each employee should be given a personnel manual that covers such issues as work schedules; office policies on smoking, dress, and telephone use; fringe benefits; sick leave; appraisals; salary increases; termination; and the grievance process. Having written

Familiarize yourself with the procedure and employee manuals and review each employee's position description to help understand individual responsibilities and how the functions interrelate.

BOX 8-1   CHECKLIST FOR A HEALTHY PRACTICE

- Physician productivity. Do you have systems in place to report various aspects of physician productivity, such as revenue generated, patient visits, and procedures done?

- Administrative productivity. Are reports or performance ratios used to assess trends in output?

- Staffing policies. Is your employee manual up to date? Does each employee have an annual performance review?

- Patient satisfaction. Have you in some way measured patient satisfaction in the past year? Are standard procedures in place for dealing with patient complaints and dissatisfied patients?

- Office procedures. Is the office procedure manual routinely reviewed and updated as needed?

- Diagnostic testing. Are foolproof mechanisms in place to be sure that abnormal screening or diagnostic test results are followed up?

- Budgeting. Does the practice have a budget, and is it used for planning and control of expenses?

- Financial reports. Do you get regular, helpful reports about practice finances?

- Employees. Are staff members cross-trained on each other's jobs? Is there a team spirit? How would you rate morale?

- Practice goals. Does the practice have a strategic plan that includes specific goals and strategies to achieve them?

work rules and practice policies helps to reduce misunderstandings about the expectations of the job. In addition, an employee manual helps ensure that the practice policies comply with relevant employee law, such as regulations governing equal employment opportunity, parental leave, sexual harassment, and the Americans with Disabilities Act (see Chapter 10).

The employee manual should contain an acknowledgment page to be signed by each employee indicating that he or she has read the manual. The signed document should be filed in each employee's personnel file.

Job Descriptions

Develop written job descriptions for each position in the practice. Each job description establishes the basic expectations of the position and helps both you and the prospective employee clarify the duties of the job and the qualifications needed to do it. In addition, the Health Insurance Portability and Accountability Act (HIPAA) security rules require that job descriptions describe the worker's needed level of access to patient health information and that the descriptions be routinely reviewed for accuracy and appropriateness. Job descriptions also should be reviewed regularly to ensure that staff members are not performing tasks beyond their licensing or training. "Boiler plate" medical office job descriptions are available and can be a good starting point, but experts advise tailoring the description to include specifics and expectations for your practice.

Compensation

Develop a salary range for each job title. Find out what salaries are being paid for comparable positions in your area and try to at least match these levels. In addition, compare the salary ranges for different positions within the practice to be sure the different levels of responsibilities are matched appropriately with the pay. Pay levels should be reviewed periodically to ensure internal equity and external competitiveness.

Employee benefits also are part of compensation. Sometimes, in lieu of higher salaries, practices can offer benefits, such as flex time, that employees greatly value but that have little direct cost to the practice.

Options for health care coverage and retirement plans have tax implications and can be complicated. It is advisable to retain a qualified consultant to help set up an employee benefits package appropriate for the size of the staff and the practice income.

Hiring

The physicians in a group practice should decide together what their roles will be in the hiring process. For example, all physicians in a small group might be involved in hiring the office manager. For hiring other nonclinical staff, the manager could handle recruitment, telephone screening, and initial interviews, with one or more physicians interviewing the two or three finalists.

There is no single right way for hiring staff—make the hiring process fit your practice. If one physician has the main responsibility for billing, for example, that physician would probably have more involvement in hiring billing and coding staff.

Throughout the recruitment and hiring process, ensure that no candidate is discriminated against. Questions about or references to the following aspects of applicants should be avoided:

- Race, age, sex, ethnic background, or religion
- Medical history or disabilities
- Club or organization memberships
- Physical characteristics
- Marital status
- Pregnancy status or plans
- Previous workers' compensation claims
- Political affiliation
- Union membership or affiliation
- Sexual preference
- Other sources of income

More information about discriminatory practices is contained in Chapter 10.

TIP

Always check previous employment references and verify current licensure for licensed personnel.

Supervision

Regularly let your staff know how they are doing. Any performance problem should be identified and discussed when it occurs, and documentation of this discussion should be kept in the employee's personnel record. Tell the individual explicitly what changes to make in behavior or performance of duties and convey confidence that improvement will be made. When the employee does improve, comment on it positively.

The following principles are helpful in day-to-day supervision:

- Do not speak or act in haste. Especially when offering criticism, take time to think your comments through—do not offer off-the-cuff reactions.

- Give employees regular opportunities to comment on the practice operations, and be open to their perspectives. Ask how they are doing and what you can do to help them do their jobs more effectively. If an employee asks for something you cannot give, explain why, and probe to learn what the real goals of the individual are. (See Chapter 7 for more information on negotiating and conflict resolution.)

- Be specific. A generality such as "you are doing a great job" has its place, but it is better to point to a specific action for praise or criticism.

- Be wary of acting on hearsay. It is unfair and usually unproductive to tell someone "Others have told me . . ." or "Your co-workers are concerned. . . ." Take time to find out what happened and ask for the employee's side of things.

- Focus on the behavior, not the individual.

- Do not avoid confrontation, even though it may be uncomfortable. If someone is disruptive, habitually late, or performing poorly, deal with it. Ignoring it demoralizes the good employees.

TIP

Offer praise in public and criticism in private.

Evaluations

An appraisal system provides a planned means of communicating with employees in a nonconfrontational way about how they are performing. Evaluations also provide the documentation necessary to support actions such as promotion, termination, and bonuses. Establish a standardized process and written format so that all employees are evaluated consistently. All staff should receive performance reviews at least annually.

The performance review process should include the following components:

- Standards for measurement

- Review of performance in achieving goals

- Identification of the employee's strengths and weaknesses

- Setting goals and timelines for improvement

- Opportunity for the employee to comment

Do not wait until "review time" to give employees feedback about their performance. If an individual has been supervised appropriately, the annual review should not contain any surprises. Moreover, if an employee's performance is not satisfactory and you have not commented on it, you have implicitly conveyed that the performance is acceptable.

TIP

Immediate feedback, both positive and negative, is the most effective form of performance appraisal.

Training and Resources

Establish a standard orientation program for new employees. Health Insurance Portability and Accountability Act rules require training on patient health information privacy and security procedures as part of the initial employee orientation. Records of such training must be maintained for 6 years.

Develop ways for your staff to be trained on each other's jobs as much as possible. Cross-training not only provides for back-up when an employee is absent or needs additional help, but also contributes to team building within the practice.

Make sure staff members have the reference tools they need, such as current information on coding, HIPAA, and Medicare compliance. In addition, make available relevant articles and books for staff development, such as resources about patient satisfaction, office efficiency, and career development.

Continuing education and training help to keep staff performance at its best. Funding classes and training courses for employees is a good way to show your appreciation for your employees and your interest in furthering their job and career goals.

Efficient Operations and Patient Flow

Pay attention to the details of practice operations. Efficiency in the office affects patient perceptions of your practice, staff morale, and the cost of doing business.

Procedure Manual

The office procedure manual should cover the daily operations of the practice. It should be separate from the employee handbook. Procedures should be updated regularly, and each should show its effective date and date of last revision. Consultants suggest retaining a copy of revised policies for 10 years.

Place the procedure manual in each work area of the office, so each employee has ready access to it. Because written policies and procedures help reduce variation in patient care and clerical functions, a well-written and current procedure manual is an essential part of ensuring quality.

The following are topics typically covered by a procedure manual:

- Medical records (eg, documentation, retention, filing)

- Release of information

- Telephone advice

- Telephone protocols
- Appointment scheduling
- Patient registration
- Patient discharge
- Payment postings
- Closing out day and month
- Billing and collections
- Patient confidentiality
- Laboratory test protocols
- Prescription policy
- Samples of forms
- Purchasing policies

TIP

Put your procedure manual to work. Use it for training, cost control, marketing, and quality improvement.

Telephone Protocol

The procedures manual should offer clear guidelines for the staff who handle telephone calls, including how callers are greeted and how different types of calls should be handled. It should cover when calls from patients will be returned by the staff.

All telephone calls should be documented, both for medical–legal reasons and in the interest of good medical care. To facilitate such documentation, post a call disposition sheet at the front desk with categories of calls in order of importance:

1. Emergency patient
2. Urgent patient
3. Routine patient
4. Another physician
5. Pharmacy
6. Hospital
7. Personal
8. Sales and detail

Appointment Scheduling

Protocols for scheduling should be covered in the procedure manual. Incorporate the following tips for practice efficiency into your scheduling policies:

- Each physician should have input into the design of his or her own appointment schedule.

- Aim to stay on schedule. Most patients do not mind waiting for 5 or 10 minutes past their scheduled appointment time. Patients tend to associate long wait times with an uncaring attitude on the part of the physician and the staff. If patients are kept waiting for 15 minutes past their scheduled appointment times, office staff or a physician should explain the reason for the delay and offer to reschedule the appointment.

- Mix short, intermediate, and long appointments to allow more flexibility for dealing with unanticipated long patient visits and to help reduce backlogs in the reception area.

- Ensure that appointments are not scheduled too far in advance; setting appointments too far in the future can increase the "no-show" rate.

- Minimize the no-show rate by reminding patients of their appointments. Automatic calling systems are available to do this. If you lack the staff time or resources to make reminder calls, consider sending preprinted postcards.

- Establish procedures for handling walk-ins and emergencies. Be sure all physicians in the practice are aware of these procedures.

Office Space

Much detail goes into setting up and maintaining key areas of the office. In addition, your facility should comply with the requirements of the Americans with Disabilities Act (see Chapter 10 for more information).

Reception Area

The following are general guidelines for a pleasant and welcoming reception area:

- Have an area near the door to accommodate coats and umbrellas.

- Chairs with arms are more comfortable than those without.

- The decor should convey a sense of cheerfulness and well-being.

- Receptionists should be able to see the entire reception area from their workstations, but patients should not be able to overhear staff conversations.

- Reading material should be current and in good condition; in addition to magazines, provide patient education materials and practice brochures containing personal profiles of the physicians and the practice's mission statement.

- Post signs as needed, such as notices of cell phone policies or policies regarding payment when services are rendered.

Once a month, sit in your office reception area for a few minutes. Check out how comfortable the chairs are and whether the upholstery is in good condition. Are the plants healthy and the magazines appealing? Most important, make sure every aspect of the area is clean—the windows, the furniture, and the woodwork.

Restrooms

Your office should have a restroom available for patients. A staff member should be responsible for monitoring the condition of the restrooms periodically during the day. In addition, you can consider placing cards that provide telephone numbers for confidential contacts regarding abuse and other sensitive subjects in the restroom.

Examination Rooms

Examination rooms typically range in size from 8 ft by 10 ft to 10 ft by 12 ft and should be set up to accommodate a diverse range of procedures. Examination tables should be positioned to allow 360-degree access to the patient, with items needed during an examination within easy reach of the physician. Standardize these items, along with other instruments and supplies, in each examination room. One room may be designated for special equipment and procedures, such as ultrasonography.

At least two examination rooms should be available for each physician working at any given time; three rooms per physician is a better ratio, allowing one for a patient being seen, one for a waiting patient, and one being cleaned and prepared for another patient. Use a flag or light system for staff and physicians to identify whose patient is occupying which room.

Check-Out Area

The check-out desk or counter should afford privacy. This allows the patient to make payment arrangements and ask questions she may have about prescriptions or referrals.

Equipment and Supplies

The American College of Obstetricians and Gynecologists' Committee on Practice Management has developed a list of equipment and supplies needed by a new obstetric–gynecologic practice at www.acog.org. The list includes both clinical and office supplies as well as medical equipment and office furniture.

Only one individual should have responsibility for ordering supplies. This eliminates duplicate orders and allows one individual to become familiar with prices and vendors. In addition, the purchaser can monitor the rate of use and develop a schedule for ordering so rush orders are not needed.

Strategic Development and Marketing

The purpose of strategic planning is to actively move your practice toward success rather than passively accepting or responding to changes that occur around you. Developing a strategic plan serves several functions:

- It helps the partners ensure they are in agreement about the current and future scope of the practice.

- It provides a roadmap for making decisions about the practice essentials, from location and equipment to staffing skills, policies, and finances.

- It creates a tool for measuring goals for performance, growth, patient satisfaction, and other elements of practice.

Marketing is just one aspect of a strategic plan. Be aware of the distinction between marketing and selling or advertising. Marketing is the process of determining what your customers want and need from your practice and then tailoring your practice to deliver those services as effectively and efficiently as possible. Selling, in contrast, is aimed at convincing customers to use the services you offer.

Mission Statement

The first step in strategic planning is to write a simply stated mission statement that defines the purpose of your practice and how you want the practice to be viewed by your patients. For example, "We will provide compassionate, comprehensive, cost-effective, high-quality health care to women of all ages," or "Our practice will provide the highest-quality gynecology and oncology services in the metropolitan area."

Research and Analysis

The next step is to gather information about your current situation—both external and internal. Internal factors include the professional and business skills of the clinical and administrative staff, as well as the practice finances.

External factors include the demographics of the population in your service area; the competition; the resources, such as hospitals and consultants; and the third-party payers. Consider the women's health care needs of population segments that are growing or shrinking. A survey of your patients can be extremely helpful in identifying both their needs for services and their perceptions of your practice.

Build on your situational assessment by conducting an analysis of the strengths, weaknesses, opportunities, and threats related to your practice. This analysis will help you identify potential changes to make your practice more successful.

Goals

Your research identified the needs of your patients, the community, the hospital, managed care plans, and other physicians. To meet those needs, set specific goals that are measurable and achievable, with deadlines for reaching them. Some examples include:

- Decrease patient waiting time to an average of no more than 15 minutes by February 2006.

- Add a maternal–fetal specialist to the practice by July 2006.

- Return all patient telephone inquiries within 30 minutes.

- Develop an education program on menopause to use in the community beginning in April 2006.

- Participate in Greater Metropolitan Health Plan by May 2006.

Strategies

Determine actions needed to achieve your goals. The strategies should be specific, including steps involved, who is responsible for each one, and a schedule. Involve everyone in the practice in achieving the goals (see Chapter 7 for more information). You also need to budget for your strategies to ensure you have the resources needed and to estimate the return on investment.

Some strategies may help to achieve more than one goal. You may find it useful to organize strategies using the traditional "Four P's" of marketing strategies:

- Product. The services you offer to your potential customers to fill a need.

- Place. The location and attractiveness of your facility, as well as the office hours of your practice.

- Promotion. The ways in which you let potential customers know about your services, such as a patient brochure or a series of women's health workshops at a community center.

- Price. The fees you charge and discounts you offer through contracts with health plans or other means.

Sometimes it is not clear whether an activity is a goal or a strategy. For example, you may decide that you need a new computer system. This may be a strategy to accomplish an end dealing with efficiency, but it also is a goal that will require several actions to achieve. It is not important how it is categorized, as long as you get it done.

Implementation and Monitoring

Establish methods to measure progress on strategies. Use quantitative measurements as much as possible. Let everyone in the practice know what is expected regarding strategies. Use team meetings for individual reports of actions. Update the strategic plan at least annually to assess progress and redefine goals.

Quality and Productivity Review

Quality in medical practice has several components, including controlling costs, satisfying patients, and providing high-quality care (Box 8–2). To review and improve quality, you need to have ways to define, measure, and monitor aspects of each component.

Continuous quality improvement is the process of setting measurable standards, collecting data, identifying system problems, making corrections, and collecting new data to see if the problem has been fixed. A successful quality improvement program must be ongoing—the "continuous" of continuous quality improvement.

Develop definitions of desired outcomes and ways to measure them. Be wary of focusing a great deal of effort on improving a process without affecting outcomes.

BOX 8–2   AREAS TO MONITOR FOR QUALITY IMPROVEMENT IN THE OFFICE

- Medical records and information systems
- Appointments and scheduling—patient flow
- Patient relations
- Patient communications
- Telephone communications
- Personnel management
- Equipment and drugs
- Complications and adverse outcomes

Data from American College of Obstetricians and Gynecologists. Guidelines for women's health care. 2nd ed. Washington, DC: ACOG; 2002.

The entire staff—clinical and nonclinical—must be active in providing input, implementing changes, and evaluating results. Patient input also is a critical component of quality improvement.

Your practice will benefit from ongoing review of quality and productivity, and your efforts also will pay off with managed care plans, which often ask for documentation of such activities. Be prepared to demonstrate your quality-review activities, such as medical record reviews, use of treatment protocols, patient surveys, and minutes of team meetings related to quality improvement.

Patient Surveys

Patient surveys can be useful both for strategic planning and quality improvement. You can use a survey to assess patient needs and wants and also to measure changes in their satisfaction with your services. You can use a practice consultant to conduct the survey for you, purchase preprinted surveys to send and tally yourself, or develop your own survey questions.

Develop an initial survey to provide a baseline. In subsequent surveys, repeat a core list of questions to compare responses. You can add a few new questions each time to find out about special topics of interest.

To make the survey results most useful to you, include two questions on each subject. One question assesses their satisfaction with something: "How satisfied were you with the amount of time you spent in the reception area?" The second question helps establish priorities: "How important is it to you that you see the doctor within 20 minutes of your scheduled appointment?" By combining the responses to these questions, you can weigh the issues to address—areas that reflect low satisfaction and high importance.

Monitoring Productivity

One tool to evaluate your practice's effectiveness is the use of performance ratios. A performance ratio expresses the relationship between two amounts. This relationship can be expressed as a fraction, a percentage, or a decimal.

Performance ratios most often are applied to practice finances, but they can be developed for every operational area of the practice (see Chapter 9 for more information on using ratios to monitor financial performance). Physicians in the practice should monitor and compare their productivity, using measures such as the Resource-Based Relative Value Scale, patient visits, or income generated. Examples of performance ratios that measure productivity are shown in Table 8–1.

The best use of these ratios is to monitor trends within your practice. Comparing ratios between medical practices, even obstetric–gynecologic practices, can be misleading because of differences in location, patient base, specialization, and other variables (see Chapter 9 for more information about outside comparisons).

Computer Systems

A checklist for information technology considerations is shown in Box 8–3. A principle of determining information technology needs is to consider software applications first. The software dictates what hardware you need. In addition, your computer system must have protective software, such as virus scanning and protection from spyware programs, to comply with the HIPAA Security Rule (see Chapter 10 has more information about HIPAA requirements).

The first step is to define the functions you want to computerize. Include current operations as well as changes anticipated over the next 5 years. Experts suggest that your system has approximately a 5-year life before it is obsolete. If you are upgrading an existing system, identify the deficiencies that need correcting.

Practice Management Systems

Most practice management software packages contain applications for the following functions:

- Registering patients
- Making appointments, including generating a call list for reminders

Table 8–1. Productivity Performance Ratios

Performance To Be Monitored	How To Calculate Ratio	Comments
Physician productivity	Procedures, patient visits, or examinations divided by number of full-time physicians	Use a similar formula for each physician or for specific procedures
Physician revenue	Net revenue divided by total number of full-time physicians	—
Office staff per physician	Number of full-time support staff divided by number of full-time physicians	—
Office staff productivity	Net revenue divided by total number of nonclinical staff	Use a similar formula for specific areas of productivity, such as office appointments per receptionist

BOX 8-3 **CHECKLIST OF INFORMATION TECHNOLOGY CONSIDERATIONS**

- Cost. Installation of hardware and software, supplies, maintenance, upgrades
- Vendor. Years of experience, financial stability, obstetric–gynecologic clients
- Ease of operation. Switching between accounts and menus, simplicity of commands, time needed for account set-ups and look-ups
- Flexibility for modification. Ability to accommodate changes
- Options for restricted access. Use of passwords for different functions
- Report generation. Inclusion of details you need or ability to customize
- Maintenance, backup, and service. Experience of technicians, schedules for service and upgrades
- User support. Availability both online and by telephone, speed of response
- Training. How long, where offered
- Customization. Percentage of products with custom options, cost and time needed to complete

- Generating bills
- Posting payments
- Transmitting claims to insurers
- Creating various financial reports
- Generating reports of current procedural terminology and diagnostic code usage, by physician and overall

These applications should be integrated so that, for instance, the user making an appointment can easily pull up the patient's financial data. Increasingly, practice management software programs also provide connections and applications for interacting with laboratories and pharmacies.

If you have managed care contracts, you may want to consider additional functions, such as:

- Electronic data interchange technology to communicate with the plans' systems

- Ability to specify approved facilities and procedural and diagnostic codes
- Categorization of preauthorization requirements for services defined as "required," "recommended," or "not required"
- Ability to define limits for charges and number of visits for each plan
- Generation of reports on activity by provider, such as Medicare resource-based relative-value scale profiles or other productivity measures
- Creation of cost and revenue reports based on procedural codes and relative value units
- Ability to customize the referrals for various plans' requirements (period of time, dollar amount, number of visits, or treatment plan)
- Issuance of warning when contract limits for referrals are approached
- Alerting for referrals that require authorization
- Ability to maintain membership logs, including identifications and start and termination dates
- Ability to post capitation payments and track payments by member count (even if you currently are not capitated, you may be in the future)

Electronic Medical Records

The technology for electronic medical records is changing rapidly as more practices are computerizing, and systems vary widely in the functions they provide. The following tasks can typically be done with the more sophisticated electronic medical record systems:

- Record history, physical, and notes of patient visits
- Prescribe medications
- View laboratory test results
- Communicate electronically with staff

Successfully implementing an electronic medical records system requires commitment from all of the group physicians to make the change. In addition to the financial investment, it takes time for individuals to feel comfortable with the new system. Consultants say you should expect implementation and training to cost up to one third of the total electronic medical records outlay. The investment in training is essential; without it, the conversion to an electronic medical records system will fail.

Experts also recommend phasing in the implementation, starting with nurses and office staff. Physicians should wait to use the electronic medical records system until the rest of the staff is using the system efficiently.

The expectation is that electronic medical records systems will be integrated with practice management systems in the future. This means, for instance, that when you order a diagnostic test, you can find out what insurance the patient has and whether her plan requires preauthorization. Two-way data flow between the practice management data and the electronic medical records is a feature to look for if you are installing an electronic medical records system.

In evaluating an electronic medical records system, look for flexibility in data entry, with options such as voice recognition, typing, using a stylus, and even handwriting. The system should allow customization of built-in templates, forms, or checklists.

Physicians in the group should decide if they want to work together to create one common medical record template that all will use or whether each physician will create his or her own template. In some obstetric–gynecologic practices, the physicians have worked together to create a uniform template for obstetrics because they cover for each other on obstetrics, but each physician has customized his or her own template for gynecology.

E-mail With Patients

Electronic communication with patients offers many advantages but should not be done using regular e-mail. A secure e-mail system will allow you to send and receive patient messages with special provisions for authentication, encryption, and protection by a firewall (Box 8–4).

In a secure e-mail system, the patient must enter a user identification and password, both for sending and receiving messages. She is notified in her regular e-mail when you have posted a message to her on the secure system. Secure e-mail programs that comply with HIPAA privacy rules are available from several vendors and also can be integrated into your practice web site.

Physicians have been reluctant to use e-mail with patients because of concerns about security, liability, and lack of reimbursement. As physicians learn how these issues can be addressed, use of e-mail in practice will undoubtedly become more common. For example, some insurers are beginning to pay for consultation provided electronically under small pilot programs.

If you offer e-mail as an option to patients, be sure they understand that they should never use it in an emergency. It also is a good idea to adopt a written policy regarding electronic patient communication and to notify patients of your policy.

BOX 8–4 RECOMMENDED ATTRIBUTES OF SECURE E-MAIL

- Encrypts all communications in transit to ensure privacy.

- Permits patient communication only with providers who have accepted the patient's request for online communication.

- Allows providers to selectively block communication from certain patients.

- Prevents forwarding of messages to standard e-mail systems.

- Provides a means to control staff access to specific categories of messages.

- Provides senders with reliable means of knowing whether their messages have been delivered.

Types of Systems

Systems come in three types: 1) UNIX-based, 2) Windows-based, and 3) browser-based. Each has its benefits and drawbacks:

1. UNIX. For complex functions, experts report that UNIX is better than Windows. When an individual is manipulating data or using the computer all day, UNIX, which is entirely keyboard-based, is faster than working with a mouse in Windows.

2. Windows. A Windows-based system will be easier for schedulers and nurses who do not use the computer full time. Some Windows-based systems incorporate keyboard commands for much of the data entry, thus accommodating both the billing staff, who usually are the ones using the system non-stop, and the front-office staff.

3. Browser. A browser-based system uses an Internet browser format. The practice contracts with an "application service provider" for access to practice management programs provided at a remote site. Staff in your office use an internal, secure private network and connect to the remote site by a high-speed Internet connection. One advantage of this method is the ease of use: the browser links allow staff to jump from one function to another without having to use menus. Another advantage is the cost: the practice does not have to buy its own computer server, and the desktop terminals connected to the service provider cost a fraction of what a desktop personal computer or laptop would cost. In addition, the service provider's staff maintains the system, provides updates, and answers staff questions.

Choosing a Computer Vendor

Take time to research vendors. Attend trade shows and check out the information technology vendors exhibiting at ACOG's Annual Clinical Meeting. Search online for systems and try the online demonstrations and tutorials available. Talk to other obstetrician–gynecologists about what they have used. A key consideration is whether the software was written with obstetrician–gynecologists in mind.

Develop a Request for Proposal

Once you have identified a number of suitable vendors, send a request for proposal to at least five. Briefly describe your practice, give each an identical list of the features you want, indicate the criteria you will use to evaluate proposals, and ask for target dates for installation and implementation.

See the Product in Action

Use the proposals you receive to select approximately three vendors to demonstrate their products. Before the demonstration, prepare a checklist to evaluate each package. For any demonstration or site visit, include your practice staff who will use the product.

If you are installing an entirely new system, try to visit practices using systems similar to ones you are considering. Choose a site to contact yourself; the vendor's references will be hand-picked happy customers or may even be compensated with discounts or extra service packages.

Some demonstrations are conducted online, but if you are keeping existing hardware, the demonstration should use the equipment you have installed. Use actual data from your practice when possible.

Vendor Selection

Expect the vendor you select to help with all aspects of your system implementation: site preparation, training, data conversion, and ongoing support. Be sure the vendor is conversant with HIPAA requirements and can provide written documentation that the products you choose are HIPAA-compliant (see Chapter 10). Before signing a contract, ask an attorney to review it.

Sources of Information

General Practice Management

- *Encyclopedia of Practice Management*, published by Practice Management Information

Corporation: www.medicalbookstore.com or 800-633-7467

- *Essentials of Physician Practice Management*, published by Jossey-Bass: www.josseybass.com/wileycda or 877-762-2974

- *Fundamentals of Medical Management: A Guide for the Physician Executive*, 2nd ed., published by the American College of Physician Executives: www.acpe.org or 800-562-8088

- *Medical Economics* magazine allows free web site access to archived articles on practice management and technology: www.memag.com

- Medical Group Management Association sells books on all aspects of practice management, from personnel and operations to finances and computerization: www.mgma.com or 877-275-6462

- *Starting a Medical Practice*, 2nd ed., published by the American Medical Association: www.amapress.com or 800-621-8335

Personnel Issues

- *Job Description Manual for Medical Practices*, published by the Medical Group Management Association: www.mgma.com or 877-275-6462

- *Personnel Management in the Medical Practice*, 2nd ed., published by the American Medical Association: www.amapress.com or 800-621-8335

- Professional Association of Health Care Office Management: www.pahcom.com or 800-451-9311

- Society for Human Resource Management: www.shrm.org or 800-283-7476

Office Equipment and Operations

- "Companies That Buy and Sell Used Medical Equipment," prepared by ACOG: www.acog.org

- *Developing Ambulatory Healthcare Facilities*, a free guidebook available from the nationwide architectural firm Marshall Erdman & Associates: www.erdman.com or 800-322-5117

- "Starting a Practice—A Resource List" (includes both clinical and clerical supplies as well as medical equipment and office furniture), prepared by ACOG's Committee on Practice Management: www.acog.org

- *Telephone Triage for Obstetrics & Gynecology*, by Vicki E. Long and Patricia C. McMullen: sales.acog.org or 800-762-2264

Strategic Planning

- *Simplified Strategic Planning: A No-Nonsense Guide for Busy People Who Want Results Fast!* by Robert W. Bradford, J. Peter Duncan, and Brian Tarcy: www.amazon.com

- *Team-Based Strategic Planning: A Complete Guide to Structuring, Facilitating and Implementing the Process*, by C. Davis Fogg: www.amazon.com

Quality Improvement

- *Managing Quality of Care in a Cost-Focused Environment*, published by the American College of Physician Executives: www.acpe.org or 800-562-8088

- *Quality Health Care: A Guide to Development and Using Indicators*, published by Jones and Bartlett Publishers, Inc.: www.amazon.com

- *Quality Improvement in Women's Health Care*, rev. ed., published by ACOG: sales.acog.org or 800-762-2264

Computers

- *Automating the Medical Record*, 2nd ed., published by the American Medical Association: www.amapress.com or 800-621-8335

- *How to Select and Implement the Right Computer Solution for Your Practice:* www.medicalbusinesspublishing.com or 800-428-2310

- "List of Information System and EMR Vendors" (from the most recent ACOG Annual Clinical meeting): www.acog.org

- Medem, Inc.: www.medem.com

Chapter 9.　Practice Finances

The Physician's Role

Although you are likely to delegate the daily financial management of the practice to your practice manager and use an accountant to prepare taxes and annual financial statements, it is important to know how to monitor the overall financial health of your practice. Numerous daily and monthly reports should be generated to help you monitor the practice finances. It takes time to develop an understanding of the implications of these reports and to track trends, but attention to finances is essential for success in practice.

Your practice manager should be able to prepare a simple, one-page summary of key data about practice financial profitability and statistics you want to monitor. An outside consultant should be able to help your practice create internal reporting mechanisms.

Because the practice accounting functions and many management tasks are delegated, it is important to choose the right staff and consultants to help you, whether it is a dedicated staff member, a financial advisor, or a combination of the two. In addition to someone who can "crunch the numbers" and give you reports, look for someone who can see trends and help you plan for the growth of the practice. If you use an outside firm, most practice management experts say that it is important to find someone with experience with physician practice finances (see Chapter 3 for more information on this issue).

Budgeting

The purpose of an operating budget is to help you plan and control expenses and project revenue. Once a budget is prepared for a period, it can be used to compare actual expense and revenue to see if you are below, above, or at expectations. Used in this way, a budget can be a very important tool to identify warning signs of negative trends within the practice.

A budget can be very important, even in a small practice, if the practice is seeking a loan; it demonstrates accountability and plan-

> *Because the practice accounting functions and many management tasks are delegated, it is important to choose the right staff and consultants to help you...*

ning to a lending institution. To begin to prepare a budget, gather information and reports about expenses and revenues from the previous year.

Revenue

Your budgeted revenue is an estimate of all fees for services rendered, including hospital visits and consultations, minus any discounts given. Income from other sources, such as subleases in your facility, also should be included as separate revenue line items.

Expenses

For expenses, the amount set for each line item should be based on past expenses and a projection of any changes expected, such as price increases, changes in patient volume, and salary increases. Listed as follows are typical major categories of medical practice expenses:

- Personnel salaries
- Personnel benefits
- Payroll taxes
- Rent or mortgage
- Utilities
- Telephone
- Postage
- Laboratory
- Medical supplies
- Administrative supplies
- Insurance
- Legal and accounting fees
- Promotions and marketing

The total of these expenses is considered the practice overhead.

Controlling Costs

Annual surveys reporting average obstetric–gynecologic practice expenses in each category are available from a number of sources, such as the Medical Group Management Association. A 2003 national survey published by *Medical Economics* showed that obstetrician–gynecologists spent 57% of practice revenues on overhead expenses, more than any other specialty, in large part because of the high cost of medical liability insurance. Survey averages can help you develop benchmarks for your practice budget but should be used with caution.

TIP

Invoices should be verified against packing slips and deliveries.

Personnel

Given that people are the most important asset of a medical practice, it is not surprising that staff compensation is the biggest expense. Accordingly, it pays off to make sure you have the right number of staff doing the right things in the most efficient way.

According to Practice Support Resources, Inc., the average number of full-time employees per full-time physician in an obstetric–gynecologic practice is 4–4.5. If your staff-to-physician ratio is higher than the average, you may need to examine staff efficiency and make adjustments to staffing levels, such as number of hours worked or even eliminating a position. But remember that survey averages are just that—the average within a range. Your practice policies or patient base may justify having higher staff-to-physician ratios.

The 2003 survey of practice expenses conducted by *Medical Economics* found that nonphysician staff salaries (not including benefits) in obstetric–gynecologic practices averaged 28% of all overhead expenses. If the number of staff in the practice seems to be in line with national averages but the percentage of expenses going to salaries is high, analyze the reasons and consider if changes are warranted:

- Scrutinize overtime hours: is the appointment schedule chronically running late? What tasks are taking overtime hours to complete?

- If possible, use a lower-paid employee, such as a file clerk, to do tasks done by highly paid staff, such as nurses.

- Contact a high-school work-study program to hire a part-time student for filing and other clerical duties. Proper training and supervision are vital.

Operations

Office procedures should always be monitored for efficiency. The following suggestions are offered by management consultants for reducing costs:

- Use a postage meter. Consultants advise that this use reduces mailing costs by at least 10–20%.

- Limit express shipping.

- Use bulk mailing services when possible.

- Use annual buying agreements and buying consortiums to negotiate lower supply prices.

- Analyze tasks that are being done in-house that could be outsourced, and vice versa.

- Computerize paper processes. Hours spent managing, filing, and retrieving paper are reduced, and software applications have built-in functions that catch mistakes (see Chapter 8 for more information about computer applications).

How To Read Financial Statements

Three financial statements describe the financial status of a practice (or any organization). These are 1) the balance sheet, 2) the income statement, and 3) the cash flow statement.

Balance Sheet

The balance sheet shows the overall financial condition of the practice. It presents a financial position at a specific time, such as the end of a year. It lists the practice's assets, liabilities, and owners' equity. The balance sheet must always balance: the total assets must equal the sum of liabilities plus owner's equity. Typically, balance sheets list the assets on the left and the liabilities and equity on the right.

Assets

Assets represent the wealth owned by the practice and usually are listed in order of their liquidity— the readiness with which they can be turned into cash. The assets usually are grouped into "current assets" and "noncurrent assets." A current asset represents cash or something that could be converted into cash fairly quickly (within 1 year). A noncurrent asset is something that would typically take longer than 1 year to convert to cash, such as property. For example, assets might be listed as follows:

- Cash

- Accounts receivable

- Inventory of clinical and office supplies

- Property

- Equipment and furniture

Liabilities

The practice liabilities are the claims against the assets—an obligation the practice has to pay something. Examples of liabilities include accounts payable (unpaid bills), salaries owed, taxes due, and loans payable.

Liabilities might be grouped as current liabilities and long-term or "noncurrent liabilities." Similar to the definitions of asset categories, current liabilities are obligations that need to be paid within 1 year, and noncurrent liabilities will be paid over a period of more than 1 year.

Equity

The equity, also referred to as "capital" or "net worth," represents the amount the owners have a claim on if the assets were liquidated to pay off the liabilities. The owners' equity is that part of the assets that exceed the liabilities. In other words, it is whatever the partners own after the money owed is deducted from the assets. The equity might represent "contributed capital," money the partners have put into the practice, or "retained earnings," income that has accumulated and has not been distributed to the owners.

Income Statement

The income statement compares revenues with expenses over a short period, usually 1 month, and no more than 1 year. It totals the revenue generated by the practice and subtracts the expenses for the same period to come up with the literal "bottom line"—the net income, sometimes called earnings. The income statement is referred to by numerous other names, including statement of operations, profit and loss statement, and income and expense report.

Cash Flow Statement

The statement of cash flow or working capital shows cash income and disbursements over a period of time (Table 9–1). It begins with the cash balance at the beginning of a period, adds and subtracts income and outgo for that period, and carries over the ending balance to the beginning of the next period.

Billing and Collections

Documentation and Coding

Proper documentation of your patient services is critically important to the financial success of a medical practice. Your billing staff uses your documentation in the medical record to assign procedural (CPT-4) and diagnostic (ICD-9) codes to claims submitted for reimbursement.

You need to document your services using terminology that the billing staff can appropriately interpret to select the correct codes for the claim. If you are not familiar with coding definitions, the reimbursement process can get bogged down or, worse, inappropriate codes can be assigned, resulting in lower reimbursement, denial by the insurance company, or charges of fraud.

Many physicians think of coding issues as something the billing staff should handle, but it is your responsibility to understand the process and learn appropriate documentation so that it is done properly. Medical management consultants say that electronic records that allow point-of-

Table 9–1. Simplified Cash Flow Statement

	January	February	March	Year to Date
Entering Cash Balance	$20,237.67	$58,080.30	$75,701.33	$109,142.26
Receipts				
Fees Collected	$65,046.04	$45,078.44	$59,052.78	$169,177.26
Interest Income	$68.26	$70.12	$61.55	$199.93
Total Income	$65,114.30	$45,148.56	$59,114.33	$169,377.19
Disbursements				
Physician salaries	$12,000.00	$12,000.00	$12,000.00	$36,000.00
Administrative salaries	$8,734.17	$8,954.28	$7,299.15	$24,987.60
Employee benefits	$944.17	$967.95	$789.04	$2,701.16
Rent	$2,465.17	$2,465.17	$2,465.17	$7,395.51
Utilities	$163.92	$175.88	$155.79	$495.59
Insurance	$2,964.25	$2,964.25	$2,964.25	$8,892.75
Total Disbursements	$27,271.67	$27,527.53	$25,673.40	$80,472.60
Net Income	$37,842.63	$17,621.03	$33,440.93	$88,904.59
Ending Cash Balance	$58,080.30	$75,701.33	$109,142.26	$109,142.26

care documentation and coding significantly improve reimbursement.

The American College of Obstetricians and Gynecologists' annual publication, *CPT Coding in Obstetrics & Gynecology*, is an excellent guide to help you understand the ins and outs of coding. It explains the definitions of the level of service; required documentation of the patient's history, physical examination, and your level of medical decision making; and many aspects of coding, such as how payers define global surgical and obstetric packages.

TIP

Some insurance companies have their own definition of a "global obstetric package." Find out what services are included in the relevant carrier's package before providing services.

Billing Procedures

Sending bills to insurance companies as often as possible is an essential part of protecting the practice's revenue stream. Submitting claims daily is optimal. In addition to getting the claim in process faster, frequent billing reduces the effect that an individual event, such as a software bug or a bag of mail being lost, could have on your total revenue. If claims are batched by the week or month, such an adverse event could affect a big portion of income.

Collection Policies

Medical practice consultants suggest that the biggest problem physician groups have in managing their finances is their failure to collect what they have legitimately earned. The following typical collection policies should be spelled out in your policy manual:

- Gather correct patient and insurance information at the time of the visit.

- Ask the patient for both primary and secondary insurance information.

- At each subsequent visit, confirm the patient's address, employer, and insurance coverage.

- Collect copayments and deductibles from the patient at the time of service.

- Explain your billing procedures to patients.

- Bill for services promptly.

- Know what information payers need to pay claims.

- Post money received and adjustments to accounts daily.

- Make daily bank deposits.

Reports To Watch

The following reports can be used to monitor your billing and collections:

- Charge lag. This report shows the time (number of days) between the date a service was provided and date the claim is submitted. Shorter is better. Cash flow will improve when charges are sent quickly after services are provided.

- Aging analysis (days in accounts receivable). This report shows the outstanding monies owed to the practice, divided into categories of how old the bill is: 0–30 days, 31–60 days, 61–90 days, 91–120 days, and more than 120 days. The amounts within each category of age are further divided by payers. This report can quickly show you if certain payers take more than 90 days to pay claims.

Internal Financial Controls

Embezzlement and diversion of funds are always a possibility in business, and all businesses—including medical practices—must guard against it. An embezzler usually is a trusted employee who has the confidence of the employer. In many cases, the embezzler has been given more authority than he or she should have.

In addition to internal controls described here, the practice should have periodic audits by an outside accountant. All employees handling cash or accounting records should be bonded (see Chapter 6).

Office Procedures To Reduce Risk

Policies and procedures should be in place—and adhered to—that protect assets, ensure legal compliance, and reduce the opportunities for errors and fraud. In addition, conducting background checks and obtaining employer references are essential for every employee hired.

Segregation of Duties

Handling cash should be totally separated from maintaining records. Assign the responsibilities for the following functions to different employees:

- Opening the mail, photocopying and endorsing checks, logging in insurance and patient checks

- Posting payments, preparing bank deposit slips

- Making bank deposits

- Preparing checks for signature

- Ordering supplies

- Reconciling the checkbook

Rotation of Job Functions

Periodically reassign tasks involved with handling cash. This way no one employee is always doing the same thing.

Vacation and Leave Time

Require all employees to take vacation. Someone who is diverting cash often is reluctant to be away from work because the discrepancies might be discovered by someone covering his or her job.

Check Signing

All checks must be signed by a physician. This responsibility may be rotated among group members, and all should take the responsibility seriously.

A check should never be signed without an attached invoice. Never provide signed blank checks for the staff to fill in.

Cash Reports To Check

Several routine financial reports can be helpful in monitoring cash diversion:

- Daily Receipts. This report shows the amount and type (insurance payment, patient check, cash, or credit card) of each payment, with totals for each type. It should be checked every day against actual cash received and discrepancies resolved immediately. Running and using this report daily acts as a deterrent to theft.

- Daily Provider Activity. This report lists patient, procedure, provider, and fee charged. It should be validated against another type of practice record, such as encounter forms or a day sheet. The individual who reviews this report should not be the same individual who collects cash.

- Monthly Gross Receipts. This report shows totals of receipts for a specific month. The monthly total should balance exactly against bank deposits for the same period.

- Uncollectible Write-offs. There are several valid reasons why the amount of bad debt increases, such as an increasing proportion of managed care patients for whom the reimbursement is less than your standard fees, but increases in write-off totals also can be a sign of an embezzlement strategy in which cash payments are stolen and not recorded, so the account eventually shows up as "uncollectible."

Performance Ratios

In addition to the practice's financial statements, performance ratios are a good way to monitor practice performance. Financial performance ratios express the relationship between two amounts. This relationship can be expressed as a ratio, a fraction, a percentage, or a decimal.

Ratio analysis is another way to monitor your practice. Comparing certain ratios from month to month or even from year to year can help you identify problem areas and track growth.

A number of financial performance ratios commonly used by medical practices are shown in Table 9–2. Tracking ratios over time within your practice can tell you if you are going in the right direction.

Use caution in comparing your practice data to national averages or data from other practices. Such a comparison can be useful, but you must take into account differences in location, patient base, specialization, and practice policies. Comparative data are available from various publications as well as from numerous practice management consulting firms.

If you are using national data or even data from another obstetric–gynecologic practice as benchmarks for your practice, take the following considerations into account:

- Definitions. Check to be sure you are comparing apples to apples. For example, does

"revenue" mean net income or gross receipts?

- Reliability. Consider the source of the information and how it was collected and analyzed.

- Comparability. Look for data on practices that are similar to yours.

- Averages. Remember that means and medians are just that: they take into account the worst as well as the best. If possible, find benchmarks noted to be "best practice."

In all cases, analyze if attributes of your practice may yield financial ratios that differ from available benchmarks. For example, consider if you take more vacation time or close the office for more holidays than others or if your practice purposely pays higher-than-average salaries to

Table 9–2. Practice Performance Ratios

Performance To Be Monitored	How To Calculate Ratio	Comments
Days in accounts receivable (average collection period)	Total amount of accounts receivable divided by average daily revenue (annual revenue divided by 365)	50–65 days is a good target; more than 90 days needs prompt action.
Accounts receivable more than 90 days	Amount of receivables more than 90 days old divided by total accounts receivable	Aim for 20% or less
Collection percentage	Total receipts less refunds, divided by total charges	The closer to 100% the better; can be used for either gross or net collection ratio.
Months for accounts receivable turnover	Amount of annual receivables divided by monthly receivables	The ratio should not exceed 6 months.
Expense ratio (also called "overhead ratio")	Total operating expenses divided by net revenue	The lower the better; aim for no more than 50%.
Cost per patient visit	Total operating expenses divided by office visits during the same period	The lower the better; very useful for negotiating capitation rates.
Current ratio (liquidity)	Current assets divided by current liabilities	Most experts say a ratio of 1.5 to 1 is adequate to meet short-term debts, and 2 to 1 is recommended.
Accounts payable	Average daily purchases divided by total accounts payable	If the ratio is increasing, it is a red flag for a possible cash flow problem; it could mean that credit is being used to pay bills
Solvency (also called "debt-to-equity ratio")	Divide total liabilities by owners' equity (from balance sheet)	The lower the better; should not exceed 50%.
Profit margin	Net income divided by net revenue	Many practices like to see a minimum of 5% profit margin.

benefit from low turnover, high patient satisfaction, and high efficiency.

Sources of Information

Managing Practice Finances

- *Encyclopedia of Practice Management*, published by Practice Management Information Corporation: www.medicalbookstsore.com or 800-633-7467

- *Financial Management of the Medical Practice*, 2nd ed., published by the American Medical Association: www.amapress.com or 800-621-8335

- *Medical Economics* magazine allows free web site access to archived articles, including annual surveys of medical practices: www.memag.com

- Small Business Knowledge Base is an online source of helpful and free information for small businesses: www.BizMove.com

Financial Statements

- *A Physician's Guide to Financial Statements*, published by the American College of Physician Executives: www.acpe.org or 800-562-8088

Coding and Billing

- The American College of Obstetricians and Gynecologists Coding Workshops: www.acog.org

- *Essential Guide to Coding in Ob/Gyn*, published by ACOG: sales.acog.org or 800-762-2264

- *Frequently Asked Questions in Ob/Gyn Coding*, published by ACOG: sales.acog.org or 800-762-2264

- *ICD-9-CM Diagnostic Coding in Obstetrics and Gynecology*, published by ACOG: sales.acog.org or 800-762-2264

- *Mastering the Reimbursement Process*, 4th ed., published by the American Medical Association: www.amapress.com or 800-621-8335

- *Ob/Gyn Coding Manual: Components of Correct Procedural Coding*, published by ACOG: sales.acog.org or 800-762-2264

Embezzlement

- Employee Theft Anonymous lets employees report theft anonymously; the web site notifies the employer by e-mail: www.etheft.com

- "Preventing Embezzlement": www.bizmove.com/general/m6t1.htm

Benchmarking

- *Cost Survey*, published annually by the Medical Group Management Association: www.mgma.com or 877-275-6462

- *Industry Norms and Key Business Ratios*, published annually by Dun and Bradstreet, includes ratios for physician practices: available in the business reference section of libraries

- *Medical Economics* magazine publishes an annual survey of practice revenues and expenses, by specialty: www.memag.com

- *Physician Compensation and Production Survey*, published annually by the Medical Group Management Association: www.mgma.com or 877-275-6462

- *Practice Management STATS Quick Reference 2004*, published by Practice Support Resources, Inc: www.practicesupport.com or 800-967-7790

Chapter 10. **Laws and Regulations**

Occupational Safety and Health Administration

A number of regulations issued by the Occupational Safety and Health Administration (OSHA) apply to all medical practices, regardless of size. Other OSHA regulations apply only to facilities with 10 or more employees.

Occupational Safety and Health Administration Standards That Apply to Medical Practices

Medical practices must comply with OSHA standards for seven areas of workplace safety:

1. Bloodborne pathogens. Practices must abide by the following procedures:

    *   Establish an exposure control plan and update it annually.

    *   Use devices for protection, such as sharps disposal containers and self-sheathing needles.

    *   Enforce safety procedures, such as hand-washing and use of protective equipment.

    *   Provide personal protective equipment, such as gloves, gowns, and masks.

    *   Make hepatitis B vaccinations available free to employees with potential exposure.

    *   Provide testing and other follow-up activities to workers who have been exposed.

    *   Use warning labels and signs on storage and refuse containers.

    *   Provide information and training to employees.

    *   Maintain employee medical and training records.

2. Hazardous chemicals. Your office must have a written list of the hazardous chemicals of any kind that are stored or used.

> *A number of regulations issued by the Occupational Safety and Health Administration . . . apply to all medical practices, regardless of size.*

For each chemical, employees must have access to the manufacturer's data sheet on handling the chemical and containing spills.

3. Emergency exits. Safe exits must exist for emergencies, and easily visible evacuation diagrams must be posted.

4. Electrical use. Occupational Safety and Health Administration rules apply to the safe use and location of electrical equipment, including computers, sterilizers, refrigerators, and microwaves.

5. Reporting injuries and illnesses. Although the federal OSHA regulations exempt medical offices from keeping an injury and illness log, some states require it (Box 10–1 lists states with OSHA-approved health and safety programs). Check into your state requirements.

6. Occupational Safety and Health Administration poster. Every practice must display OSHA's poster notifying employees of their rights to a safe workplace. Free posters can be downloaded from OSHA's web site (www.osha.gov) or ordered at 800-321-6742.

7. Ionizing radiation. Practices that offer X-ray services must designate restricted areas, give employees in those areas personal radiation monitors, and post caution signs on rooms and equipment.

If the practice has a laboratory, OSHA standards for Occupational Exposure to Hazardous Chemicals in Laboratories may apply.

Other areas related to workplace safety are not regulated by OSHA, but the agency provides recommendations and links to help employers ensure a safe environment. For example, OSHA's web site includes resources related to latex sensitivity, workplace ergonomics, and workplace violence.

Free Consultation Available

The Occupational Safety and Health Administration offers a free, confidential consultation service on request. A trained professional will schedule a

---

BOX 10–1   STATES WITH OCCUPATIONAL SAFETY AND HEALTH ADMINISTRATION-APPROVED HEALTH AND SAFETY PROGRAMS*

Alaska	Michigan	South Carolina
Arizona	Minnesota	Tennessee
California	Nevada	Utah
Connecticut[†]	New Jersey[†]	Vermont
Hawaii	New Mexico	Virgin Islands[†]
Indiana	New York[†]	Virginia
Iowa	North Carolina	Washington
Kentucky	Oregon	Wyoming
Maryland	Puerto Rico	

*As of October 2004

[†]Programs cover government employees only.

---

visit to examine your operations and facility for potential safety hazards. The consultant will give you a written report and recommendations and also will provide training and help you implement the recommendations. No safety violations are reported to OSHA enforcement staff. Go to www.osha.gov/dcsp/smallbusiness/consult.html for information on the consultation service.

Clinical Laboratory Improvement Amendments

The Clinical Laboratory Improvement Amendments (CLIA) regulate laboratory testing on human specimens. If your office performs laboratory tests, it must have a CLIA certificate. (If specimens, including blood, are *only collected*, a CLIA certificate number is not needed.)

A certificate of registration and CLIA number allow physicians to operate an office laboratory and receive Medicare reimbursement. However, CLIA standards apply whether or not Medicare claims are filed.

The Centers for Medicare & Medicaid Services (CMS) runs the CLIA program, including registering laboratories and enforcing compliance. To register a laboratory in your office, complete an application (form CMS-116 available from the CMS web site at cms.hhs.gov/clia/cliaapp.asp) and send it to the appropriate agency in your state—usually the state health department or a CMS regional office.

Clinical Laboratory Improvement Amendments regulations have established three categories of tests, depending on the complexity of the test method: 1) waived, 2) moderate complexity, and 3) high complexity. The more complicated the test, the more stringent the requirements.

The CLIA program issues five types of laboratory certificates:

1. Waiver. A Certificate of Waiver allows a laboratory to perform only "waived tests," tests that are considered to be so simple that there is little risk of error or patient harm. They include pregnancy tests, fecal occult blood tests, and some urine tests. Currently, 40 tests have been approved for certificate-of-waiver status. For the complete list, go to www.fda.gov/cdrh/clia. Laboratories with a certificate of waiver have to pay a fee every 2 years and follow manufacturers' instructions for testing. These laboratories are not subject to routine surveys, but 2% of them are randomly selected for a survey as part of a quality control project begun in 2002.

2. Provider-Performed Microscopy Procedures, most commonly referred to as PPMP. This certificate permits a laboratory to perform a subset of the moderate-complexity tests. The tests must be performed by a physician or midlevel practitioner. They include wet mount preps, pinworm examinations, fecal leukocyte examinations, and urine sediment examinations. Routine laboratory surveys are not required. A PPMP certificate also permits the laboratory to perform waived tests.

3. Registration. This certificate is issued initially to laboratories applying to conduct moderate- or high-complexity tests. It permits the laboratory to perform the tests until it receives a certificate of compliance or accreditation.

4. Compliance. Laboratories performing moderate- or high-complexity tests are surveyed onsite and determined to be in compliance with the relevant CLIA standards before receiving this certificate.

5. Accreditation. An accredited laboratory goes through a process that includes an onsite survey conducted either by CMS; a state laboratory licensure program; or one of several private accrediting agencies, such as the Commission on Office Laboratory Accreditation, the College of American Pathologists, or the Joint Commission on Accreditation of Healthcare Organizations.

Health Insurance Portability and Accountability Act

The Health Insurance Portability and Accountability Act of 1996 (HIPAA) established standards to protect the privacy of personal health information. Every medical practice that conducts certain electronic transactions must comply with HIPAA's three sets of regulations: 1) transaction and code sets, 2) security, and 3) privacy.

There are stiff penalties for violations of the HIPAA regulations. A practice can be fined $100 per incident for accidental disclosure of patient health information, up to $25,000 per year. Purposeful misuses could result in fines of up to $250,000 and 10 years in prison.

TIP

Your state might have privacy or security requirements that are more stringent than those of the Health Insurance Portability and Accountability Act. Check with your state medical society or a consultant to find out how the two sets of regulations apply to your practice.

What is Protected Health Information?

Protected health information is broadly defined by HIPAA and includes patient information transmitted or maintained in any form—by electronic means, on paper, or through oral communications. Protected health information has three defining criteria:

1. It is created or received by a health care provider, health plan, employer, or health care clearinghouse.

2. It relates to the past, present, or future physical or mental health or condition of a patient; the provision of health care to a patient; or the past, present, or future payment for health care.

3. It identifies the patient or includes information that could be used to identify the patient.

Transaction and Code Sets Rule

The Transaction and Code Sets Rule (compliance date: October 16, 2002, unless the practice requested an extension to October 16, 2003) established electronic standards that vendors, insurance companies, and providers have to use for electronic claims filing and related activities, such as checking on eligibility, obtaining referrals and authorizations, and following up on claims. Health care providers are responsible for making sure the software they use and the vendors they contract with are compliant with HIPAA standards. Claims filing software must be tested for filing Medicare claims successfully. The Centers for Medicare & Medicaid Services maintains a list of HIPAA vendors (billing services, clearinghouses, and software vendors) who have tested their software successfully with Medicare at www.cms.hhs.gov/hipaa. The American College of Obstetricians and Gynecologists worked with expert consultants to develop a complete manual, *HIPAA Transaction & Code Set Standards: A How-To Guide for Your Medical Practice*, about how to comply with the Transaction and Code Sets Rule.

Security Rule

The Security Rule (compliance date: April 21, 2005) set up administrative, physical, and technical safeguards to protect patient information that is sent or maintained electronically. These regulations apply to many aspects of a medical practice, from training staff and establishing office procedures to setting up computer passwords and installing antivirus software.

Because of the wide variations in the places where it will be implemented—from hospitals to solo office practices—the HIPAA Security Rule has quite a bit of flexibility built in. Of its 41 specifications, 20 are required to be implemented by all providers and 21 are considered "addressable," which means they should be considered and implemented if they are "reasonable and appropriate" for your practice. You must document the actions taken on all 41 specifications. If you determine an addressable specification is not reasonable and appropriate, you must document why and implement an "equivalent alternative measure if reasonable and appropriate."

Following is a summary of both the required and the addressable Security Rule specifications (some have been combined):

- Designate a security officer who has final responsibility for the practice's security compliance (may be the same individual as the privacy officer).

- Analyze the risks to the confidentiality and integrity of the practice's electronic patient information.

- Establish procedures for electronic auditing, which tracks who has accessed the computer files, what was done, and when.

- Create a "workforce clearance system"—background checks on employees and use of procedures that allow access to records only to authorized users.

- Protect access to computer files through procedures such as use of passwords and automatic time-out features when a computer is idle.

- Use encryption or secure messaging to communicate with patients or vendors electronically.

- Use computer data protection programs, including antivirus software, firewalls, spyware, and back-up-and-recovery programs.

- Establish policies for reporting both accidental and intentional security incidents.

- Develop a contingency plan to protect data during emergencies, such as floods, fires, or terrorism.

- Implement business associate contracts governing information created or transmitted electronically.

- Develop policies and procedures for security of all computer workstations, including personal digital assistants and laptops, and evaluate the policies and procedures periodically.

- Train all physicians and staff.

- Establish a sanction policy that holds all staff and business associates accountable to the practice's security policies.

All of these requirements are explained in ACOG's *HIPAA Security Rule Manual: A How-To Guide for Your Medical Practice*. In addition to definitions and explanations, the manual includes sample policies and procedures and checklists.

Privacy Rule

The HIPAA Privacy Rule (compliance date: April 14, 2003) applies directly to most obstetric–gynecologic practices and regulates how you may use and disclose protected health information. Physician practices are required to:

- Notify patients of their privacy rights and your office privacy practices and obtain their written acknowledgment of receiving the notice.

- Designate a privacy officer responsible for developing and implementing privacy policies and procedures (may be the same individual as the security officer).

- Provide training to all employees about the HIPAA regulations and your practice's privacy policies and procedures.

- Make written agreements with business associates about disclosure of patient health information.

- Use or disclose personal health information only as permitted by the Privacy Rule.

- Disclose only the minimum amount of patient information necessary to achieve the purpose of the disclosure (you are not limited in your disclosures to other providers for treatment purposes).

- Permit patients to inspect and get a copy of their health information.

The Privacy Rule specifies that patients can ask to amend inaccurate medical records. You may deny the request, but you must provide a written statement explaining the reason for the denial. *HIPAA Privacy Manual: A How To Guide for Your Medical Practice,* published by ACOG, is an excellent source of the policies, contracts, and forms that are needed to comply with the Privacy Rule.

Business associates are individuals or companies that receive or create patient information from you to perform nonpatient-care services, such as billing, accounting, collecting, or consulting. You must have a written agreement with each business associate that requires them to safeguard the information.

If you do not give patient health information to the other party, a business association agreement is not needed for HIPAA requirements. For example, agreements are not needed with a janitorial service or photocopier repair service.

TIP

Situations involving disclosure of patient information to other providers for treatment of a patient do not require a business associate contract.

Employment Law

Fair Labor Standards Act

The Fair Labor Standards Act applies to virtually all employers in the United States. In addition to regulating child labor and establishing a minimum wage, the law governs overtime pay.

All employee positions must be designated either "exempt" or "nonexempt" for overtime pay requirements. Employees who are nonexempt must be paid at least 1.5 times their regular pay rate for working more than 40 hours per week. Each work week stands alone: if someone works 30 hours 1 week and 50 hours the next, you cannot average the hours for purposes of overtime pay. However, hours that an employee is out for sick leave or vacation do not count toward overtime pay because the employee was not physically on the job. You can obtain guidelines for categorizing specific positions and additional requirements of the regulations from the Department of Labor's Wage and Hour Division.

Antidiscrimination Laws

A number of federal and state laws protect workers against discrimination. Title VII of the Civil Rights Act applies to employers with 15 or more employees and prohibits discrimination because of race, religion, sex (including pregnancy), and national origin. These are discussed as follows, along with the Age Discrimination in Employment Act. The Americans with Disabilities Act is covered in a separate section because it applies both to employment and to patient services.

Most states also have antidiscrimination statutes, and some states prohibit discrimination based on additional characteristics, such as marital status, sexual orientation, or personal appearance. State laws may apply to employers with fewer than 15 employees.

Antidiscrimination laws and regulations cover virtually all aspects of employment—job advertisements and recruitment, interviewing and hiring decisions, compensation, promotion, firing, and retirement plans. Details of the regulations, including rules for documentation, retention of records, and required workplace posters, are available from the Equal Employment Opportunity Commission (EEOC).

Sexual Harassment

Title VII of the Civil Rights Act protects workers from sexual harassment and gives the employer responsibility for the conduct of others—both employees and nonemployees, including patients and vendors. Although the federal law applies only to businesses with 15 or more employees, many states have laws covering sexual harassment that apply to more employers.

The courts have recognized two basic types of sexual harassment. The first is "quid pro quo" harassment where a supervisor conditions employment, compensation, or promotion on the employee's submission to sexual advances. The second is "hostile environment" sexual harassment in which sexually oriented conduct creates an offensive and unpleasant working environment.

Following are examples of conduct found by the courts to be illegal sexual harassment:

- Repeated sexual innuendo, off-color jokes, and lewd remarks

- Letters, notes, e-mail, and graffiti of a sexual nature

- Sexual touching, propositions, insults, and threats

- Sexually oriented demeaning names

The EEOC encourages employers to clearly communicate to employees that sexual harassment will not be tolerated and to establish an effective complaint process. Employers are required to take immediate and appropriate action when an employee complains. Experts in this field recommend developing written policies regarding sexual harassment, including the complaint process and sanctions, and conducting a training session to sensitize employees and communicate your policies.

Pregnancy Discrimination Act

Pregnancy Discrimination Act, an amendment to Title VII of the Civil Rights Act, prohibits discrimination against women affected by pregnancy or related conditions. It regulates hiring practices and work during pregnancy and maternity leave and requires equal treatment regarding health insurance and fringe benefits offered by an employer.

Women affected by pregnancy or related conditions must be treated in the same manner as other applicants or employees with similar abilities or limitations. For instance, if an employee is temporarily unable to do her job because of pregnancy, she must be treated the same as any other temporarily disabled employee.

Age Discrimination

The Age Discrimination in Employment Act protects individuals who are aged 40 years or older from employment discrimination based on age. The regulations protect both employees and job applicants and apply to employers with 20 or more employees (this differs from Title VII of the Civil Rights Act, which has a threshold of applicability at 15 workers).

Although the law does not specifically prohibit asking an applicant's age or date of birth, the EEOC closely scrutinizes requests for age information because such inquiries might deter older workers from applying or might indicate intent to discriminate. Similarly, a job application should not ask for dates of military service or school graduation; these can be considered proxies for inquires about age. Details about requirements of the age discrimination law are available from the EEOC.

Equal Pay Act

In addition to Title VII, the Equal Pay Act prohibits compensation discrimination based on sex. The Equal Pay Act was passed in 1963 as an amendment to the Fair Labor Standards Act. The law requires employers to pay men and women equally for equal work performed in the same establishment under similar conditions. Because it is part of The Fair Labor Standards Act, the Equal Pay Act applies to most employers, regardless of size.

Family and Medical Leave Act

The Family and Medical Leave Act affects employers with at least 50 employees. It requires employers to allow eligible employees to take job-protected, unpaid leave for up to 12 weeks in a 12-month period for any of the following reasons:

- Birth, adoption, or foster-care placement of a child
- Care of a child, spouse, or parent with a serious health condition
- A serious health condition of the employee

The law also requires employers to continue group health benefits coverage during the leave. After completion of the leave, the employee must be restored to the same or an equivalent position.

Details about the regulations are available from the Department of Labor's Wage and Hour Division. Many states also have laws regarding family and medical leave that may differ from the federal law.

Americans with Disabilities Act

The Americans with Disabilities Act (ADA) cuts a wide swath—it prohibits discrimination in public accommodations, employment, transportation, government services, and telecommunications. Americans with Disabilities Act regulations regarding employment discrimination apply only to employers that have 15 or more employees. The regulations for public accommodations apply to all physician offices.

To offset costs of complying with ADA regulations, small businesses can take a tax credit of up to $5,000 per year; a tax deduction of up to $15,000 per year is available to all businesses for barrier removal and alterations.

The EEOC has responsibility for enforcing the employment provisions of the ADA. The Department of Justice handles complaints about other ADA violations.

Americans with Disabilities Act Regulations About Employment

Employers with 15 or more employees are prohibited from discriminating against "qualified individuals with disabilities." A qualified individual with a disability is an individual who meets the requirements of a job and can perform the "essential functions" of the position with or without reasonable accommodation. If someone is qualified to do the job except for limitations caused by a disability, you must consider if making "reasonable accommodation" would enable him or her to do the job.

Who is Protected

An individual is considered to have a disability if any of the following criteria apply:

- Current physical or mental impairment. The impairment must substantially limit a major life activity, such as seeing, hearing, speaking, walking, breathing, performing manual tasks, learning, caring for oneself, and working. A minor short-term condition, such as a sprain, broken limb, or the flu, would not be covered.

- History of such an impairment. Individuals are protected by the ADA if they have a record of a disability, such as an individual who has recovered from cancer or mental illness.

- Perceived disability. Individuals who are regarded as having a substantially limiting impairment, even though they may not be functionally impaired, fall under the definition of a protected individual.

In addition, the ADA protects individuals discriminated against because they have a known association or relationship with certain individuals. For example, someone who works as a volunteer with patients who have acquired immunodeficiency syndrome (AIDS) is protected from biases an employer may have about that association.

Reasonable Accommodation

The ADA uses the term "reasonable accommodation" to describe a modification to a job or the work environment that will enable an applicant to participate in the application process or enable an employee to perform essential job functions.

Examples of reasonable accommodation include making your office readily accessible to an individual with a disability, restructuring a job, modifying work schedules, and buying or changing equipment. You are not required to make an accommodation if it would impose an "undue hardship," meaning that it is excessively costly or disruptive to your practice.

Americans with Disabilities Act Regulations for Public Accommodations

The ADA requirements regarding accessibility and communication apply to all facilities open to the public. Therefore, they are the ones that are most likely to affect physician practice.

Accessibility

New facilities must be built to be accessible to individuals with disabilities, and existing buildings must be modified when it is "readily achievable," meaning it can be done "without much difficulty or expense." Retrofitting buildings to be fully accessible is not possible or required for every business. The Department of Justice and the Small Business Administration, which provide guidance to businesses, point out that much can be done without much difficulty or expense to improve accessibility. Examples are installing a bathroom grab bar; lowering a paper towel dispenser; rearranging furniture; installing offset hinges to widen a doorway; or painting new lines to create an accessible parking space.

Regarding leased office space, the ADA gives the landlord and tenant joint responsibility to remove barriers or provide auxiliary aids. The landlord and tenant may decide by lease agreement who will actually make the changes, but both remain legally responsible.

Communication

To communicate effectively with hearing-impaired patients, the ADA requires you to provide auxiliary aids, such as sign language interpreters, assisted listening devices, notetakers, written materials, television encoders, and telecommunications devices for the deaf. You are expected to consult with the patient who has the disability about her needs before acquiring a particular aid or service.

The law does not require you to provide an aid or service that would be an "undue hardship" to your practice. Although the cost sometimes may exceed your fee for treating the patient, this alone is not considered an undue hardship—you are expected to consider it part of the cost of doing business.

Undue hardship is defined as an action that is excessively costly, extensive, substantial, or disruptive or that would fundamentally alter the nature or operation of the business. Factors to consider include the cost of the aid, financial resources of the provider, and the difficulty of locating or providing the aid.

Limited English Proficiency

Although the ADA does not require services for patients with limited English proficiency, this topic is included here because its provisions are similar to those of the ADA communications requirements. Title VI of the Civil Rights Act requires physicians who receive Medicaid or State Children's Health Insurance Program reimbursement to take adequate steps to provide language assistance to patients with limited English proficiency.

The type of assistance that must be provided to meet this requirement depends on factors such as the size of your practice and the frequency with which particular languages or patients with limited English proficiency are encountered. The Office of Civil Rights investigates complaints about possible noncompliance. If accommodating patients with limited English proficiency would be so burdensome that it would be difficult for your practice to stay in operation or if there are alternatives for patients to have access to the type of services you provide, the Office of Civil Rights will not find your practice noncompliant.

Antitrust

Federal antitrust laws have existed since 1890 and are designed to protect competition. Violations can result in severe penalties and even criminal

prosecution. The Department of Justice and the Federal Trade Commission are charged with enforcing antitrust laws.

Generally, you must not collaborate with physicians outside your own practice about fees, discounts, boycotts, or other actions that would restrain trade or competition. Following are examples of activities that could violate antitrust laws:

- Agreeing with competing physicians about increasing fees by a certain percentage or charging interest on past due accounts

- Jointly threatening a boycott of a health maintenance organization or insurance company

- Agreeing with competing practices on "market allocation" arrangements—dividing up the territory where you will promote your practice

The legal role of physicians in negotiating with managed care plans has been an issue of concern since the 1990s. Legislation has been passed in some states allowing physicians to negotiate collectively, and several physician advocacy groups, including the American Medical Association, have supported bills introduced in Congress to afford relief from the restrictions on joint physician negotiating.

In 2004, the Federal Trade Commission and the Department of Justice released a 300-page report repeating their position that collective bargaining by independent physicians would have a negative impact on health care competition. This area is in a state of flux as physicians look for legal ways to gain leverage with managed care plans. If you are involved in collective negotiations of any kind, you should seek legal counsel to avoid antitrust implications.

Stark Laws

Two sets of federal laws, known as Stark I and Stark II, prohibit referring Medicare or Medicaid patients for certain health services if you or an immediate family member have a financial relationship to the service. (The laws get their names from their main legislative sponsor, Representative Fortney "Pete" Stark.)

If you submit a Medicare bill in violation of Stark regulations, penalties include fines of up to $15,000 for each service plus twice the reimbursement claimed, and you may be barred from participating in Medicare and Medicaid. A violation of the Stark law occurs when all of the following elements apply:

- You refer a Medicare or Medicaid patient to a health care entity in which you or an immediate family member has a financial interest.

- The referral is for one of a list of designated health services.

- No Stark-rule exception applies.

To ensure you do not unintentionally violate Stark regulations, it is important to know how these terms and entities are defined in the regulations. The key points are briefly defined as follows.

Designated Health Services

Stark specifies the following categories of health services as subject to restrictions on referrals:

- Clinical laboratory services

- Physical therapy, occupational therapy, and speech-language pathology services

- Radiology and certain other imaging services

- Radiation therapy and supplies

- Durable medical equipment and supplies

- Prosthetics, orthotics, and prosthetic devices and supplies

- Home health services

- Outpatient prescription drugs

- Inpatient and outpatient hospital services

- Parenteral and enteral nutrients, equipment, and supplies

Definition of Financial Relationship

A financial relationship means having a direct or indirect ownership or investment interest in another entity or receiving compensation—again, directly or indirectly—from an entity. Such entities include hospitals and other organizations providing any of the designated health services.

The interpretation of indirect compensation can be subtle. If a hospital recruits you and gives you an incentive bonus or other monetary relocation package, it would be a Stark violation if any of the following conditions apply:

- The compensation is contingent on referrals or establishing exclusive privileges at that hospital

- You are required to refer patients to the hospital

- You are barred from establishing staff privileges at another hospital

As long as the relocation incentive is not tied to referrals, it is not in violation of Stark.

Definition of Immediate Family

The usual definition of immediate family includes parents, spouse, children, and siblings. In addition, the Stark definition includes inlaws, grandparents, grandchildren, stepparents, stepchildren, stepsiblings, and stepgrandparents.

Exceptions

Some of the most significant exceptions to Stark violations include:

- Physician services given by or supervised by a physician in the same group as the referring physician

- Some in-office ancillary services when certain location, supervision, and billing requirements are met

- Services furnished to enrollees of prepaid plans

- Certain services that are subject to frequency limitations under Medicare rules, including screening mammography and ultrasound bone density measurement

- Compensation from an entity to a physician that is based on fair market value of the services and not on the volume or value of the referrals

Medicare Billing Fraud

A number of federal laws address misrepresentation of health care claims. The prohibition against filing false claims applies to individuals who "know or should know" that the services were not provided as claimed. The HIPAA regulations further clarified that there need not be proof of specific intent to defraud to prove that someone is in violation of this law.

A false claim is one in which any statement made to secure reimbursement is inaccurate. Thus, claims with even minor infractions—mistakes in dates, provider numbers, or place of service, for example—could be considered false under this broad definition. Generally, such individual clerical mistakes are not of great concern to regulators. Instead, they look much more closely at patterns of behavior.

The most common forms of Medicare fraud include:

- Billing for services not provided
- Misrepresenting the diagnosis to justify payment
- Soliciting, offering, or receiving a kickback
- Unbundling or "expanding" charges
- Falsifying certificates of medical necessity, treatment plans, or other medical records to justify payment
- Submitting duplicate reimbursement claims
- Upcoding—billing for a higher-level procedure than the one actually provided

Penalties

Physicians who have gone through it say that a Medicare audit or investigation is an extremely traumatic experience. In addition, the financial consequences of an investigation can be devastating. The penalties that can be assessed for fraudulent claims range from $2,000 to $10,000 per improper item on the claim form plus triple your original charge. In addition to these penalties, violators also can be excluded from the Medicare program for a set period.

Develop a Practice Compliance Plan

Your practice should develop and maintain a Medicare compliance plan—written rules and procedures to reduce any chance of wrongdoing, such as improperly billing Medicare. Such a plan is not required by law, but having one in place is helpful if you are audited. Most important, the plan serves as an internal tool to establish clear policies for filing claims and teaching staff and physicians about compliance. A compliance program is meant to ensure that you and your staff will not inadvertently, negligently, or intentionally engage in illegal activity.

Seven steps are suggested by the U.S. Department of Health and Human Services Office of the Inspector General for an effective compliance program:

1. Develop standards and procedures. Establish a commitment to compliance and outline expectations for billing and coding, patient care, documentation, and payer relationships.

2. Designate someone with oversight responsibilities. A high-level individual should oversee development and enforcement of the compliance plan. This compliance officer should have authority to implement compliance procedures in all areas of the practice, regardless of his or her role in the practice.

3. Conduct effective training. Cover compliance procedures during training for all new employees. Further, training for coding and billing staff should be conducted at least annually. Be sure to document all meetings and retain copies of agendas and attendance sheets.

4. Develop lines of communication. Create a mechanism for employees to report suspected violations—anonymously, if possible. The system also should protect complainants from possible retaliation.

5. Create monitoring and auditing systems. Audit bills and medical records for compliance with billing, coding, and documentation requirements.

6. Investigate problems and take disciplinary action. Set up a system to consistently investigate allegations of improper activities. Potential sanctions range from oral warnings and written reprimands to demotion, temporary suspension, and termination.

7. Respond to offenses and initiate corrective action. If a practice discovers credible evidence of its own possible violation, it must report such conduct to the appropriate government agencies. In a governmental audit, such prior reporting will be in your favor and generally will reduce the penalties.

Sources of Information

Occupational Safety and Health Administration

- Occupational Safety and Health Administration: www.osha.gov or (202) 693-2220

- *Health & Safety Management for Medical Practices*, published by the American Medical Association: www.amapress.com or 800-621-8335

Clinical Laboratory Improvement Amendments

- Clinical Laboratory Improvement Amendments: www.cms.hhs.gov/clia

- Commission on Office Laboratory Accreditation: www.cola.org or 800-981-9883

Health Insurance Portability and Accountability Act

- Health Insurance Portability and Accountability Act: www.hhs.gov/ocr/hipaa

- "HIPAA Consult" series in *Medical Economics,* available free in the magazine's searchable archives: www.memag.com

- *HIPAA Policies & Procedures Desk Reference,* published by the American Medical Association: www.amapress.com or 800-621-8335

- *HIPAA Privacy Manual: A How-To Guide for Your Medical Practice,* published by ACOG; it comes with a CD-ROM with model policies, contracts, and forms that can be customized for individual practices: sales.acog.com or 800-762-2264

- *HIPAA Security Rule Manual,* available free to members of ACOG: www.acog.org/departments/practice/SecurityManual.doc

- *HIPAA Transaction & Code Set Standards: A How-To Guide for Your Medical Practice,* developed for ACOG members and available free online: www.gatesmoore.com/transaction_&_codesets-standards.HIPAA.ACOG.html

Americans with Disabilities Act

- Americans with Disabilities Act: www.ada.gov

- The American College of Obstetricians and Gynecologists' Committee Opinion No. 202, *Access to Health Care for Women with Physical Disabilities,* available to ACOG members: www.acog.org

- "Assisting Hearing Impaired and Non-English Speaking Patients," developed by ACOG: www.acog.org

Limited English Proficiency

- Information and technical assistance: www.lep.gov or (202) 307-2222

Employment Law

- Department of Labor Wage and Hour Division: www.wagehour.dol.gov or 866-487-9243

- Equal Employment Opportunity Commission: www.eeoc.gov or 800-669-4000

- Office for Civil Rights: www.hhs.gov/ocr or (202) 619-0805

- *The American Bar Association Guide to Workplace Law: Everything You Need to Know About Your Rights as an Employee or Employer,* published by the American Bar Association: www.ababooks.org or 800-285-2221

Stark

- American Health Lawyers Association has numerous analyses and publications: www.healthlawyers.org

- Centers for Medicare & Medicaid Services provide a summary of the law and physician resources: www.cms.hhs.gov/medlearn/refphys.asp

Medicare Billing Fraud

- *Health Care Fraud and Abuse: A Physician's Guide to Compliance,* published by the American Medical Association: www.amapress.com or 800-621-8335

- *Medicare Compliance Manual 2005,* published by Practice Management Information Corporation: www.medicalbookstore.com or 800-633-7467

- "OIG Compliance Program for Individual and Small Group Physician Practices," published by the U.S. Department of Health and Human Services Office of the Inspector General: http://oig.hhs.gov/authorities/docs/physician.pdf

Chapter 11. Personal and Professional Growth

Physician Roles

As a physician, you have opportunities and responsibilities that can take you in many directions. There are numerous avenues you can pursue that can enhance your career while offering personal enrichment.

The health care system is complex, and physicians have a unique and valuable role within that system. High-quality, effective health care delivery does not just happen. Your contributions are important not only as a provider of care but also through your involvement in such activities as policy making, peer review, teaching, mentoring, and leading.

Achieving Balance

As you develop your practice and plan your career, it is important to maintain a balance between professional responsibilities and your personal life. Take time to explore ways that you can responsibly and enjoyably expand your professional horizons without becoming burdened.

Your chosen career is demanding and can easily strain family and social bonds that you need for support. It is not uncommon for physicians to devote so much time and energy to patients that they neglect the individuals who matter most to them. Always remember there is more to life than medicine.

Managing Stress

Stress comes with the territory of being a physician, and you need to find ways to relax and keep joy in your life and your practice. Following are tips to reduce stress:

As you develop your practice and plan your career, it is important to maintain a balance between professional responsibilities and your personal life.

- Take care of yourself. Maintain a healthy weight, exercise regularly, and get enough sleep.

- Stay connected to your family. Schedule regular times to spend time together. Call your siblings and parents. Share good news and the struggles and challenges you have.

- Return to an old hobby or start a new one. Maybe you used to play a musical instrument or collect fossils. Find something you enjoy and turn to it for relaxation.

- Confide in others. Turn to someone you trust—a former professor or medical school classmate, or a professional skilled in listening.

- Set boundaries. You may need to change your hours, your patient load, or the number of committees you are on. Learn how to say "no" and feel okay about it.

- Keep a journal. Writing about what is going on around you and how you feel can help clarify issues, provide an emotional outlet, and provide a mechanism for contemplation.

Hospital Activities

Taking a leadership role in medical staff and obstetric–gynecologic department activities can have a profound and positive effect on your practice and daily professional satisfaction. The hospital's internal structure and its position in the community offer a ready-made network for you to push for enhancing women's health care. Your hospital may already have robust women's health programs in which you can support or take a leadership role. For example, obstetrician–gynecologist input and direction is vital in education about menopause, breastfeeding, and prenatal care as well as screening and referral programs, such as those for depression, domestic abuse, obesity, or smoking cessation.

Department Committees

A good place to start active involvement is within your hospital obstetric–gynecologic department, which likely has committees on education, credentials, or quality improvement. Serving as a peer reviewer in your department is an excellent way to gain a broader perspective on approaches to medicine as well as contribute to the improvement of patient care.

The American College of Obstetricians and Gynecologists' manual, *Quality Improvement in Women's Health Care,* is targeted to obstetrician–gynecologists who are involved in hospital quality improvement activities. It covers developing a departmental quality improvement program, assessing clinical competence (which is particularly helpful for credentialing activities), and screening tools to use.

Women's Health Expertise Needed

The organizational structure of the hospital administration and the medical staff—not to mention the politics of both—can be complex and take time to figure out. You may want to start by volunteering to serve on an existing hospital committee. Examples include patient safety, credentials and qualifications, operating room, physician well-being, utilization management, continuing medical education, graduate medical education, privilege denial appeals panels, and ad hoc task forces on matters such as bed allocation and length-of-stay reduction.

Working with a hospital committee is a great way to learn about how the administration and other departments function. It is an orientation to the players and the politics and can help you decide where it is most worthwhile to put your energies—what you are most interested in and where the biggest needs are.

Accreditation Compliance— Be a Team Player

Hospitals must expend a tremendous amount of effort to ensure that they meet the standards of the Joint Commission on Accreditation of Healthcare Organizations and, sometimes, other accrediting organizations. You have a responsibility, along with every member of the medical staff, to ensure compliance with the accreditation standards that apply to your practice. These range from requirements for disaster preparedness to use of abbreviations in documentation and patient orders.

Unfortunately, physicians are all too often indifferent or simply aggravated by the need to comply with accreditation requirements. There may be a widespread perspective that "it is not my problem." This attitude often leads to hostility between the hospital administration and the medical staff, which creates a climate that is not in either party's best interest, and certainly not in the patients' best interests.

Whether your institution has worked past this and has positive energy going between the physicians and administration or a negative and likely dysfunctional atmosphere exists, you can contribute positively. Your participation in committees, as mentioned previously, is one way you can help your hospital meet its accreditation requirements. In addition, you should consistently attend to paperwork, completing documents, such as those listed as follows, accurately and promptly:

- Patients' admission history and physical examination

- Informed consent forms

- Daily progress notes

- Operation and delivery dictations

- Discharge summaries

- Completion requirements for medical records, including signatures

Community Involvement and Service

The opportunities you have to do satisfying volunteer work are virtually endless. These experiences can be especially gratifying when you combine your expertise as an obstetrician–gynecologist with other activities you enjoy.

If you like to write, for example, offer to prepare a short piece on a focused topic in the newsletter of an organization to which you belong. A community newspaper also may be interested.

If public speaking is your forte, there is no end to the groups who would appreciate a talk on a relevant topic. Such opportunities are not limited to women's groups. Pregnancy-related topics, obesity, smoking cessation, or teen pregnancy prevention are a few examples of many subjects in which mixed groups would be interested.

There are numerous kinds of ongoing programs that need the involvement of obstetrician–gynecologists. Fetal and Infant Mortality Review is local and involves regular monthly meetings with a team in your community, whereas both the Indian Health Service program and international programs call for a period away from home.

Fetal and Infant Mortality Review

Fetal and Infant Mortality Review is a local process in which an interdisciplinary review team examines cases of deaths of infants aged 1 year or younger. The team meets monthly and reviews de-identified case information, including an interview with the mother. The team considers all aspects of each case—medical issues, family support, social environment, and hospital and community factors—and works to identify psychosocial and economic factors and barriers to care that affected the family during pregnancy and the infant's life. The team's findings are used to develop strategies and interventions to decrease the number of infant deaths.

Physician participation on Fetal and Infant Mortality Review teams is important. Physicians not only interpret medical information for other team members but also help open doors in hospitals, health departments, and other institutions.

Indian Health Service

The American College of Obstetricians and Gynecologists has a program in which obstetrician–gynecologists provide services to Native American or Alaskan Native women for brief periods. Assignments are available only when a hospital asks for help, often for coverage for the local obstetrician–gynecologist during leave for vacation or education. When ACOG receives such a request, the staff contacts you or another obstetrician–gynecologist who has volunteered to see if you are available and interested. Minimum service periods range from 3 to 4 weeks. The duties during this period of service include labor and delivery (especially for high-risk patients), gynecologic surgery, general obstetric and gynecologic outpatient clinic coverage, and telephone consultation to smaller hospitals and clinics.

International Outreach

Obstetric–gynecologic services are greatly needed in the developing world, where your contribution can have a profound impact on the lives of individuals and the entire community. Doctors Without Borders and dozens of other groups work to place physicians in medically disadvantaged communities all over the world.

The American College of Obstetricians and Gynecologists maintains a directory of these organizations with details about the duration of service, language requirements, and services needed. Some groups focus on clinical practice whereas others focus on educating the local health practitioners.

You can peruse this directory—divided into secular and religious groups—at www.acog.org. You also can sign up to receive an update about global opportunities: send an e-mail to majordomo@linux.acog.com and type "subscribe international" in the body of the message.

Professional Societies

Involvement in professional societies offers physicians more than collegial interaction, education, and helpful practice information. More importantly, through professional societies physicians can help define the future of medicine.

Opportunities abound for meaningful involvement and leadership development through active participation in medical societies and associations. They also give discounts to their own members on books and continuing medical education programs and typically offer members-only resources on their web sites.

Local Medical Societies

County and state medical societies usually are affiliated with the American Medical Association (AMA) and represent physicians before Congress and state medical boards, as well as other state and federal regulatory and administrative bodies. They keep members informed of policy and legislative changes in medicine, assist physicians with problems involving government agencies and third-party payers, and may provide free legal information and contract review services.

Specialty Societies

Many states, counties, and large cities have obstetric–gynecologic societies that sponsor education for obstetrician–gynecologists and support lobbying efforts on behalf of women's health. The American College of Obstetricians and Gynecologists' state sections typically work with their sister obstetric–gynecologic societies on these issues and often hold joint conferences and educational programs. Organizations representing obstetric–gynecologic subspecialties, such as maternal–fetal medicine, also offer advocacy, develop guidelines for practice, and provide advanced education.

The American College of Obstetricians and Gynecologists

Eligibility for Fellowship in ACOG begins with your certification by the American Board of Obstetrics and Gynecology. You should apply for Fellowship as soon as you become eligible.

Among ACOG's many programs are providing extensive patient education materials, developing guidelines for clinical practice, offering education and practice assistance to obstetrician–gynecologists, and publishing *Obstetrics & Gynecology*. You can get a lot more out of ACOG, however, than taking advantage of its broad array of educational materials, conferences, and publications. The American College of Obstetricians and Gynecologists offers numerous opportunities for you to take on leadership responsibilities.

A good place to start is as an officer of an ACOG section—the state-level organization of ACOG. Attend an ACOG meeting or contact one of the officers in your state and tell him or her you would like to get involved. Officer contact information is available on ACOG's web site.

Another excellent way to become involved in ACOG is through legislative advocacy. Joining the ACOG key contact program puts you in the loop to receive insider information and updates.

The American College of Obstetricians and Gynecologists also provides training for leadership. A 2-day conference, *ACOG Future Leaders in Ob-Gyn,* has sessions on a number of essential leadership skills, from decision making and managing complaints to financial aspects of an organization and working with the media.

Legislative Advocacy

Legislation and policy decisions at the local, state, and national levels affect your practice, your patients, and your community. Make an effort to learn about the legislative issues that are important to women's health care and medical practice. Policy makers and legislators repeatedly point out that they rely on thoughtful input and explanations about health care issues from physicians and other experts.

State Legislation

The American College of Obstetricians and Gynecologists monitors state legislation in all 50 states and works with Fellows in state sections to help them build coalitions, promote women's health issues, and influence health policy and legislation. Many state ACOG sections have their own lobbyist who collaborates with physicians on strategies and represents them in the statehouse and state legislature.

The American College of Obstetricians and Gynecologists' web site (www.acog.org) is an excellent place to start to learn about key issues being addressed at the state level, such as professional liability reform, contraceptive equity, physician credentialing, and perinatal human immunodeficiency virus (HIV) testing and counseling. The web site explains ACOG's positions on issues and offers talking points and strategies for approaching policy makers.

Following are some ways to get involved in state legislative initiatives:

- The American College of Obstetricians and Gynecologists. Contact the officers of your ACOG state section.

- State medical societies. State associations have active legislative departments and lobbying efforts focused on health policy and legislation. They are eager for physicians to become involved.

- Special interest groups. If you have a special interest in a specific issue, whether it is domestic violence, preterm births, or medical education, check out the web sites of related organizations. National coalitions, consumer groups, and foundations (such as the March of Dimes) often have robust legislative advocacy programs and plenty of ways for you to get involved.

Federal Legislation

The American College of Obstetricians and Gynecologists monitors federal legislation and lobbies on the behalf of obstetrician–gynecologists and women's health. Its web site posts up-to-date news, including the congressional voting records on issues of interest to obstetrician–gynecologists. In addition, the government relations portion of ACOG's web site has an action center that gives talking points and will automatically e-mail, fax, or mail your message to the office of your representative or senators.

These are two ongoing ACOG programs that offer good ways for you to engage:

1. Key Contact Program. The American College of Obstetricians and Gynecologists' key contacts are spokespersons for ACOG at the local level, providing expert information on obstetric–gynecologic issues to members of Congress. As a key contact, you receive regular e-mail updates about ACOG's legislative priorities.

2. Annual Congressional Leadership Conference. This 3-day workshop is held

every spring in Washington, DC. The conference presents timely information through small, interactive sessions and features speakers from Congress, the administration, and the lobbying community. On the third day, the conference participants visit their representatives or senators on Capitol Hill.

OB-GYNs for Women's Health

OB-GYNs for Women's Health is a nonprofit advocacy organization created by ACOG specifically to lobby for women's health interests on Capitol Hill. It created the first national obstetric–gynecologic political action committee that can help elect individuals to Congress who support legislation that improves the quality of and access to women's health care.

You can join the organization at www.physiciansforwomenshealth.org. Members of ACOG also can join OB-GYNs for Women's Health through their annual ACOG dues statement.

Patient Safety and Professional Liability

Patient safety and professional liability are being singled out because for the foreseeable future these issues will be top priorities in health care. These topics need your attention, whether in your daily patient care activities, legislative advocacy, patient education, or medical society involvement.

Tremendous energy and resources are being applied to these issues. They are being addressed through ACOG and AMA initiatives, American Board of Obstetrics and Gynecology certification requirements, hospital committees, Joint Commission on Accreditation of Healthcare Organizations accreditation, and residency training guidelines, to name just a few.

Patient Safety

Patient safety hurtled to the top of public scrutiny following the 1999 release of the Institute of Medicine's report, *To Err is Human*. Health care and legislative leaders responded by reexamining

many components of health care delivery and launching activities to address them.

Most leaders in this field have pointed to the need for system changes in all aspects of health care, from training of health care professionals to delivering care. A system is needed that has processes to prevent errors from occurring and to learn from them when they do occur. Moving from a culture of blame to a culture that encourages open discussion of errors is a key element in changing the system.

The opportunities for involvement and leadership in patient safety are extensive. At a minimum, you should be aware of your hospital's patient safety requirements that apply to your patient care, such as those about disclosing errors, reporting sentinel events, use of abbreviations, and protocols to prevent wrong site or wrong procedure surgery. Contact your hospital's risk management or quality assurance personnel to find out about relevant policies and disseminate the information to other department members.

Take the lead in incorporating patient safety protocols in your office practice. The National Patient Safety Foundation, founded by the AMA and other health care organizations, has resources you can use and numerous initiatives in which to get involved.

In the hospital environment, ensuring patient safety demands understanding the differing perspectives across a spectrum of stakeholders. For example, it is important for physicians and administrators to appreciate the role each plays in error reduction and to work together to find common ground. Your interaction with the nursing staff requires a similar approach. (See Chapter 7 for more information about becoming involved in patient safety activities.)

Professional Liability

Professional liability, always an important issue in obstetrics–gynecology, became a critical issue as the liability insurance market collapsed—first in a few hot spots and now virtually nationwide. As numerous ACOG leaders have pointed out, our liability system is broken, and profound changes need to be made.

Both ACOG and the AMA have initiatives addressing medical liability. Among the resources offered by the AMA are a Physician Action Kit and a compendium of facts supporting medical liability reform. Check the AMA web site (www.ama-assn.org) for the latest updates. Legislative advocacy and ACOG involvement, addressed in previous sections represent additional ways you can address professional liability issues.

Sources of Information
General Professional Development

- *Continuing Professional Development of Physicians: From Research to Practice*, published by the AMA: www.amapress.com or 800-621-8335

- *Strategic Career Management for the 21st Century Physician*, published by the AMA: www.amapress.com or 800-621-8335

Balance and Stress Reduction

- Center for Professional Well-Being: www.cpwb.org or (919) 489-9167

- *Medical Marriage: Sustaining Healthy Relationships for Physicians and Their Families*, published by the AMA: www.amapress.com or 800-621-8335

- *Resilient Physician*, published by the AMA: www.amapress.com or 800-621-8335

Hospital Activities

- American Medical Association Organized Medical Staff Section: www.ama-assn.org

- "Physicians Taking the Lead: 10 Ways for Hospital Physicians to be Effective Agents of Change," published by the American College of Physician Executives: www.acpe.org/leadingedge/Oct_2004_Vol1_No3/change.htm

International Outreach

- The American College of Obstetricians and Gynecologists' directory of international organizations that need physician volunteers: www.acog.org

- *Improving Birth Outcomes: Meeting the Challenges in the Developing World*, published by the Institute of Medicine: www.nap.edu or 888-624-8373

- *Reducing Birth Defects: Meeting the Challenge in the Developing World*, published by the Institute of Medicine: www.nap.edu or 888-624-8373

Professional Organizations

- The American College of Obstetricians and Gynecologists: www.acog.org or 800-673-8444

- American Association of Gynecologic Laparoscopists: www.aagl.com or 800-554-2245

- American College of Osteopathic Obstetricians and Gynecologists: www.acoog.com or 248-332-6360

- American Institute of Ultrasound in Medicine: www.aium.org or 800-638-5352

- American Medical Association: www.ama-assn.org or 800-621-8335

- American Society for Colposcopy and Cervical Pathology: www.asccp.org or 800-787-7227

- American Society for Reproductive Medicine: www.asrm.org or (205) 978-5000

- American Urogynecologic Society: www.augs.org or (202) 367-2403

- Canadian Medical Association: www.cma.ca or 800-457-4205

- North American Menopause Society: www.menopause.org or (440) 442-7550

- North American Society for Pediatric and Adolescent Gynecology: www.naspag.org or (215) 955-6331
- North American Society for Psychosocial Obstetrics and Gynecology: www.naspog.org or (202) 863-2570
- Society for Maternal-Fetal Medicine: www.smfm.org or (202) 863-2476
- Society of Gynecologic Oncologists: www.sgo.org or (312) 644-6610
- Society of Gynecologic Surgeons: www.sgsonline.org or (314) 251-6881
- Society of Obstetricians and Gynaecologists of Canada: www.sogc.medical.org or 800-561-2416
- National Medical Association: www.nmanet.org or (202) 347-1895

Legislative Advocacy

- The American College of Obstetricians and Gynecologists' Government Relations Department: www.acog.org
- OB-GYNs for Women's Health: www.physiciansforwomenshealth.org or (202) 314-5798

Patient Safety

- *Crossing the Quality Chasm: A New Health System for the 21st Century,* published by the Institute of Medicine: www.nap.edu or 888-624-8373

- *Health Professions Education: A Bridge to Quality,* published by the Institute of Medicine: www.nap.edu or 888-624-8373
- *Leading a Patient-Safe Organization,* published by Health Administration Press: www.ache.org/hap.cfm or (301) 362-6905
- *Medical Error and Medical Narcissism,* published by Jones & Bartlett: www.amazon.com
- National Patient Safety Foundation: www.npsf.org or (703) 506-3280
- *Partnering with Patients to Reduce Medical Error: Guidebook for Professionals,* published by the American Hospital Association: www.ahaonlinestore.com or 800-242-2626
- *Quality Improvement in Women's Health Care,* published by ACOG: sales.acog.org or 800-762-2264

Professional Liability

- The American College of Obstetricians and Gynecologists' Medical Liability Reform Action Center: www.acog.org
- American Medical Association Physician Action Kit: www.ama-assn.org
- *Red Alert—A Resource for Working with the Media,* published by ACOG: Request free copy at 800-673-8444, ext 2560, or e-mail communications@acog.org

Chapter 12. **Personal Finances**

Financial planning is important whether you are young or old, rich or debt-ridden. Keeping track of your finances is the starting point. The accessibility of records and documentation of expenses are essential for handling your taxes and will put you in a good position to begin financial planning. Organize files—and know where they are—for all of your finance-related paperwork (eg, loans, credit card statements, bank statements, insurance policies, and employment contracts.

Maintaining financial information electronically can be very helpful. A simple spreadsheet program can be used to list and add up your financial data, create a budget, and maintain information needed for taxes, investments, and other purposes.

If you are interested in doing more in-depth analyses and computerizing financial transactions, several software programs are available that can help you do this. The two most popular programs for money management are Intuit's Quicken and Microsoft Money. These programs have a planning feature that relates your current finances to your long-term goals—such as retirement—factoring in inflation, taxes, and investment return. Other features include checkbook management; tax preparation; and numerous analyses, such as whether to lease or buy a car.

Insurance protection is a basic element of your financial picture. You should have both life and disability insurance, as well as professional liability coverage. The amounts of insurance you carry will vary depending on your individual and family situation (see Chapter 6 for details about insurance).

> *Organize files—and know where they are—for all of your finance-related paperwork . . .*

Debt Management and Saving

Before you can plan your investment strategies for other financial goals, you need to get control of debt and create an emergency savings fund. Physicians are particularly likely to have debt problems because they start out with a huge education debt load.

Emergency Reserve

Financial advisors suggest that you should focus on building an emergency fund before paying off your debt. Otherwise, if a big bill comes in, such as a car repair, you would have to add it to your credit card, thus worsening your debt situation. The possibility of being disabled through an accident or illness is another reason it is essential to have an emergency fund because disability insurance payments usually do not begin for 3–6 months.

Most advisors suggest maintaining a 3–6-month cash reserve. Enough money for a shorter period is reasonable if you have a spouse with an income or home equity that you could use for a loan.

To find the money to put toward savings, start a spending record to see where your money is going. You can use a financial software program or simply make a worksheet. Create separate columns for two types of nondiscretionary expenses: 1) fixed expenses, such as rent or mortgage, insurance, and loan payments; and 2) variable expenses, such as essential clothing, car maintenance, food, and household utilities. In a third column list discretionary expenses, such as additional clothing, beauty care, credit card interest and fees, entertainment, household help, recreation, and gifts. In the variable expense category, be specific. Break down the purchases on your credit card so you know what category they fall into.

Analyze the totals—particularly the variable expenses—to see where to cut back on spending. Set specific monthly goals for these cut-backs, and put that money into savings.

Save some money every month toward your emergency fund. The best way to be sure this happens is to designate an amount to be automatically deposited into a savings or investment account before you receive your payroll check. If your payroll department cannot handle this type of deposit, set up an automatic transfer from your checking account to your savings or investment account.

Credit Card Debt

Interest payments make credit card debt a special problem. The following warning signs indicate credit card debt problems:

- You rarely pay more than the required minimum on credit cards.

- You make partial or late payments.

- You have to wait until payday to pay bills, or worse—you have to use cash advances from your credit card to pay.

- You have more than two or three major credit cards.

- You are at or near the credit limit on your cards.

- Each month you charge more on your cards than you pay.

- You bounce checks.

- You and your partner argue about money frequently.

- You do not know your total debt balance.

- You have been denied credit, asked to obtain a co-signer, or failed to qualify for the lowest financing rate available for a home or car loan.

If you experience some of these signs of problems, tackle credit card debt as a priority. There are some actions to take to help you get in control. The goal is to completely eliminate credit card balances and pay off the entire balance of new charges every month.

If you have more than one credit card, work first on paying off the one with the highest interest rate. Pay more than the minimum payment each month. If possible, transfer the balances on higher-interest-rate cards to a card with a lower rate.

You may find it helpful to work with a credit counselor to help you create a plan to do this. The Federal Trade Commission offers excellent advice about choosing a reputable credit counselor at www.ftc.gov/bcp/conline/pubs/credit/fiscal.htm.

Some credit counseling services use deceptive practices and scams, so it is worthwhile to know the potential pitfalls and misrepresentations. For example, a reputable credit counseling agency should give you free information about itself and the services it provides without requiring you to provide any details about your situation. If a firm does not do that, consider it a red flag and go elsewhere for help.

Agencies that belong to the National Foundation for Credit Counseling or the Association of Independent Consumer Credit Counseling Agencies must subscribe to a code of ethics, offer a low fee structure, and use trained counselors. These national organizations can give you a referral to a local agency.

Student Loan Consolidation

Consolidating your student loans into one new loan may lower the interest rates you pay. It also will combine the payments into one monthly payment and lock in an interest rate, so your monthly payments will never go up.

Having just one payment to make each month is more than just a convenience. Being late with a payment goes on your credit record; if you are repaying five or 10 different loans, missing the payments 1 month puts five or 10 bad marks on your credit record.

There are possible disadvantages of loan consolidation. These include paying more total interest over time by extending the repayment period and paying a higher interest rate on the consolidation loan than on one or more of the individual loans.

Terms To Know

If you have student loans, there are some terms you should know:

- Grace period. Period after graduation when you do not have to make loan payments. For federally subsidized loans, interest is not charged during this period, but for unsubsidized loans interest does accrue during the grace period.

- Deferment. A 12-month period when your loan payments are suspended for various reasons, such as economic hardship, military service, or graduate fellowship. Deferment is granted for 1 year at a time, after which you must reapply. Subsidized loans do not charge interest while the loan is deferred, but unsubsidized loans do.

- Forbearance. A temporary suspension or reduction of your monthly loan payments. Borrowers may qualify for forbearance if they are unable to make loan payments because of certain types of financial hardships.

Assess Your Loan Situation

Check your regular mailings about your school loans to determine the types of loans you have. Separate the public from the private loans. By law, federal loans cannot be consolidated with private ones. If you have both private and federal loans, you will need two separate consolidation loans. You should determine the status of your loans, such as whether they are in grace or deferment.

Federal Loan Consolidation

For federal loan consolidation, the timing of when you consolidate can make a big difference in your interest rate. If you consolidate your loans during the grace period following graduation, you can get an additional discount of 0.6% in the interest rate, so that is an incentive to consolidate during that period.

If you are out of the grace period, consider waiting to see what the next annual interest rate will be. Federal student-loan interest rates change once a year on July 1. The rate is tied to the final rate set in May on the 91-day U.S. Treasury bill. You may want to wait until May to see what the new rate will be. If it will increase after July 1, finalize the consolidation before then. If it will decrease, wait until after July 1. In either case, get your application paperwork done ahead of time.

The Department of Education's web site at www.loanconsolidation.ed.gov is a good place to start to determine your eligibility for loan consolidation. The American Medical Association-endorsed Collegiate Funding Services (www.cfsloans.com/ama) also has information and resources for loan consolidation and borrowing that is geared to physicians. Both of these web sites offer an online calculator that will show you what your interest rate and monthly payments would be for the loans you wish to consolidate.

Private Loan Consolidation

Financial advisors strongly suggest that you consolidate federal loans before consolidating private ones because the interest rate for federal loan consolidation is fixed and not tied to your credit score. Once you have consolidated your federal student loans, your debt-to-income ratio will improve, giving you a better overall credit score. This will enable you to secure a more favorable interest rate for your private student loan consolidation.

Some private lenders do not offer consolidation. Call the lender that services your loan to find out if it does. Be sure to ask to speak with a loan officer in the consolidation department; some individuals have been given inaccurate information from other loan officials, who may not be familiar with consolidation options. If the lending institution does not offer consolidation, you can shop around for another lender. Collegiate Funding Services has a private loan consolidation program, as do most major banks.

Only student loans are eligible for these consolidation services. Credit card balances or other general loans are not eligible.

Consolidating Loans With Those of Your Spouse

If you and your spouse both have student loans, you are probably better off to consolidate them separately. If one of you dies or becomes permanently disabled, the spouse will be obligated to pay the balance, whereas an individual consolidation loan balance is forgiven in the case of death or disability. In addition, a consolidated debt cannot be broken up in the case of divorce, and both parties continue to be responsible for the entire balance.

Shop Around

Lenders are eager to get your business and many offer appealing features, including:

- Slightly lower interest rates (approximately one quarter percent less) if you sign up to have payments made automatically
- A discount for paying on time every month for a period of years (usually three or more)

Be sure to check out any related fine print. For example, the discount for several years of on-time payments may be forfeited and not eligible for reinstatement if you obtained a legitimate deferment during that period.

Financial Plans for Specific Goals

Once you have established an emergency reserve, you should continue to invest. Where you invest your money will depend in part on when you plan to use it. In other words, set the goals first, then develop the strategies. For example, you may have goals for retirement, a vacation home, a college fund, and an annual trip to Europe. The investment strategies for each of these goals will be different.

College

As a first step, calculate what it will cost for your kids' college education. Numerous web sites, such as www.collegeboard.com, have online calculators that use basic information, such as follows, to compute how much to save each month:

- Tuition and expenses
- Years of college expected
- Years from now until college starts

The calculators will take into account the effect of inflation, the return on your investments, and tax implications. If you prefer, your financial advisor will work with you to do the calculations for how much you need to save.

Two tax-free investment plans offer good ways to save for your children's college education: 1) Section 529 plans and 2) Coverdell Education

Savings Accounts. The money earned on your investments in these plans is not subject to federal tax when you withdraw it for qualified education expenses.

Section 529 Plans

All 50 states and Washington, DC, now have Qualified Tuition Programs, known as "Section 529 plans" after the section of the Internal Revenue Code governing their requirements. There are two basic types of Section 529 plans:

1. Prepaid tuition plan. The prepaid plans specify the colleges where the money must be used—usually certain state schools. Contributions today are guaranteed to cover tuition costs in the future. In some state plans, the funds cover room and board as well as tuition.

2. Savings plan. A 529 college savings plan is an investment account, but you cannot completely control where your funds are invested. Instead, you must choose from the ones designated by each state. Some states have only a few options and some have more than 20. The federal tax exemption on withdrawals from the 529 savings plans expires in 2011. It is likely Congress will extend the tax exemption, but it is not a sure thing.

Each state has its own rules for its Section 529 plans, so check out such details as how the funds may be used, contribution deadlines and limits, tax-deductibility of your initial contributions, and the ability to transfer the account to another beneficiary. Two web sites that offer links to plans in each state are www.collegesavings.org and www.savingforcollege.com.

Coverdell Education Savings Account

The Coverdell Education Savings Account allows for tax-deductible contributions of up to $2,000 per year per student. The funds in a Coverdell account also can be used for elementary or secondary school expenses, including school uniforms and transportation.

The Coverdell plan is available only to individuals who earn less than $110,000 (or $220,000 for joint tax filers). However, if you exceed those income limits, you can give the money to your child to open an account in his or her own name.

You can choose the investment instruments for the funds, such as stocks, bonds, or mutual funds. A possible drawback to a Coverdell Education Savings Account is that the funds transfer to the beneficiary at age 18 years, allowing your "student" to use the money for something besides education. An advantage of the Coverdell Education Savings Account, in addition to the tax deduction on the contribution, is that the funds can be transferred to a 529 plan without penalty. The Motley Fool financial education web site (www.fool.com/college/compare.htm) offers an excellent side-by-side comparison of the requirements and benefits of the Coverdell Education Savings Accounts and the Section 529 plans.

Retirement

The sooner you begin saving for retirement, the better, because your contributions will have a longer time to accrue interest. A typical feature of retirement investment accounts is that you do not have to pay annual income taxes on the interest earned on the funds in the retirement account. The tax is deferred until you withdraw the funds after retirement. This arrangement generally is advantageous because most individuals are in a lower tax bracket after retiring. Most plans have penalties if you withdraw funds before a set age. Your eligibility for various retirement plans depends on such criteria as your total income, whether you are employed or independent, and whether other pension plans are available to you or your spouse.

The rules for contributions and withdrawals and the tax benefits of each vehicle are varied and complex. Moreover, the specifics of retirement plans, such as the eligibility requirements, the maximum contributions, and the tax benefits, are subject to change every year as tax laws change.

The National Association of Personal Financial Advisors offers good explanations of retirement plans and strategies in the "Consumer Services" section of its web site (www.napfa.org). Check out the Internal Revenue Service web site (www.irs.gov/retirement) for more details about specific requirements and limitations of the following retirement plans:

- Individual retirement account (IRA). An individual retirement account is an individual savings account that you can set up at a bank, credit union, or other investment organization. It allows tax-deferred contributions each year up to a limit ($3,000 in 2004) if you meet certain eligibility requirements. Even if the money you put in an individual retirement account is not tax-deductible, investing there has the advantage that the interest on the funds invested is not subject to income taxes until the money is withdrawn.

- Roth individual retirement account (Roth IRA). If your income is below a certain threshold, you can contribute to a Roth individual retirement account. Whether or not you are covered by an employer's retirement plan is irrelevant. Contributions to a Roth individual retirement account are not tax deductible, but investments in the account grow tax-free. Thus, when you withdraw funds from a Roth IRA at retirement, you do not have to pay taxes on any of it.

- Simplified employee pension (SEP). This is a special type of individual retirement account that can be established by your employer or by you if you are self-employed. If you qualify, you can make tax-deferred contributions of 25% of your annual income into a simplified employee pension, up to a maximum of $41,000 (2004 limits).

- 401(k) or 403(b). To participate in either of these plans (named for sections of the Internal Revenue Code), you must be employed by an organization that offers them. (The main difference is that 403[b] plans may be offered only by educational or charitable organizations.) As with an individual retirement account, the interest on the funds in a 401(k) or 403(b) account are not subject to federal income taxes until the funds are withdrawn. The maximum amount you can contribute as an employee is limited ($14,000 in 2005).

- Savings incentive match plan for employees (SIMPLE). This type of individual retirement account is a vehicle that small employers can set up. It allows you to divert some of your compensation into retirement savings (up to $9,000 in 2004). Your employer makes a matching or nonelective contribution. To be eligible, you cannot have any other retirement plan.

- Keogh plan. Also known as a qualified retirement plan, a Keogh plan is for self-employed individuals or small businesses. Generally, it can be set up with features like those of corporate pension plans, such as profit-sharing or defined benefits. It allows you to make tax-deferred contributions of 25% of your annual income, up to a maximum of $41,000 (2004 limits).

In planning a retirement fund, some of the following general guidelines are accepted by most experts:

- To keep your standard of living during retirement, plan for an income that is approximately 70–80% of your income before retiring. This percentage can vary, depending on your lifestyle, home ownership, and other variables.

- Put away enough retirement savings to support you to age 85 or 90 years.

Although the future of Social Security is uncertain now, you should obtain your Personal Earnings and Benefits Statement from the Social Security Administration to help determine the amount of assets you will need in retirement. You can request it online at www.ssa.gov or call 800-772-1213.

A number of online calculators are available to determine how much you need to save to reach your retirement goal. Your financial planner also can help you crunch the numbers. *Money* magazine has an easy-to-use retirement calculator at www.money.cnn.com.

Do your own research or consult with an investment advisor about how best to allocate the funds in your retirement account. Generally, the allocation depends on your personal tolerance for risk combined with how many years you have until retirement. Your retirement fund should be balanced, meaning you allocate certain percentages of the funds into different types of investments. Be sure to review your plan regularly and rebalance it as needed.

Recreation and Short-Term Goals

As with any kind of financial goal, planning for shorter-term goals starts with deciding how much money you will need and when. Once you have determined the goal, invest funds sufficient to meet it, and be sure the assets are of the type that can be converted to cash when you need it.

Estate Planning

To determine what happens to your finances when you die, you need a will. Many young physicians do not think they need a will because they have few assets or even a negative net worth. However, if you die without a will, state law determines the distribution of your estate and can drag out the process.

A will designates to whom your assets will be distributed and names an executor to handle the administration of the estate. Perhaps most important, if you have minor children, your will is the appropriate vehicle to name a guardian to raise your children. If you are married, each spouse has a separate will, and each will has provisions for guardianship of children if you should both die at the same time.

In addition to a will, you should have a living will, a health care power of attorney, and general power of attorney. These legal instruments spell out your wishes in case you become incapacitated.

Trusts can be used to gain significant tax advantages and to simplify or avoid complications of probate, which is the process that establishes the legal validity of wills. An estate planner can help you analyze whether setting up a trust will be a useful way of handling your assets.

Executing a will is not a one-time act. You should review it periodically to be sure it continues to reflect your wishes as well as any relevant changes in your life, such as marriage, divorce, or birth of children.

Advisors

Professional advice can help you in numerous aspects of financial planning and management. Refer to Chapter 3 for advice on selecting an advisor, including criteria to look for and questions to ask when checking references.

The personality of you and your advisors should mesh, whether fast-paced or laid-back, conservative or bold. Rapport and trust are essential: a financial advisor not only knows about your debts and total money picture, he or she knows about such personal issues as your values, perspective on life, and dreams.

Personal Financial Planner

Not every physician needs or wants to use a financial planner. Some physicians have the time and inclination to learn about financial management and develop plans for themselves. Others are not interested in it—or do not want to take the time to learn—and prefer using professional expertise.

Generally, a financial planner works with you to define your personal and financial goals, needs, and priorities. The planner analyzes the financial information you provide to assess your current situation and identify any problem areas or opportunities, including risk management needs, investments, taxes, and retirement and estate planning. Finally, the planner prepares a financial plan, providing projections and recommendations tailored to meet your goals and objectives, values, temperament, and risk tolerance.

In addition to accomplishing those tasks, a professional financial planner can sometimes bring other advantages to the table:

- Objectivity. A planner may see that achieving your goals according to your schedule is unrealistic. He or she might even question the necessity of some goals.

- Insight into financial complexities. A planner understands how the financial moves you might consider are interrelated, especially in light of tax implications.

- Level-headedness. A financial planner can keep you from making impulsive decisions, such as selling low when the market dips.

- Mediation. If you and your life partner have different attitudes toward money management, you may need a third party to help develop a budget or a plan that you both can live with.

A planner's services are not free. In deciding whether to use a planner, you must decide if the benefits outweigh the costs.

Financial planners charge either by commission or by a set fee. The National Association of Personal Financial Advisors supports the fee-only approach.

Fee-only advisers can set fees in different ways. They may charge an annual percentage of any money you invest with them, charge a flat or hourly fee, or charge a fee that combines those two approaches. A typical charge from a fee-only planner is 1% of the first $500,000 to $1 million of assets they manage for you. The percentage decreases as the amount of assets increases.

Commission-only advisers do not charge a fee. Instead, they are paid from the commissions on load funds or individual stocks.

Your first meeting with a planner should be free and should not focus on only one aspect of your finances, such as insurance or investments. Be wary of a planner who rushes you toward a fabulous deal or wants you to change your investments without good reasons.

Lawyer

For drawing up your will and related estate documents, you may want to use a lawyer who specializes in estate planning. See Chapter 3 for information about fees and the pros and cons of different kinds of law firms.

Accountant

As suggested in Chapter 3, when choosing an accountant, try to find one who has worked with physicians. A good accountant should be able to do more than crunch the numbers and prepare your tax returns. Expect information about the tax consequences of investments and changes in the tax law that could affect your holdings.

Insurance Agent or Broker

Look for an insurance representative who is interested in you and your family and will be with you for the long run. Financial advisors often recommend that you use an independent agent or a broker rather than an agent who works for a single company. This is based on the perception that independent agents have broader experience and may be less biased.

An exclusive agent, also called a "direct writer," is one who works for a single, big insurance company (such as MetLife, Prudential, or State Farm) and sells proprietary products. An exclusive agent might be a salaried employee, work on commission, or get some combination of salary and commissions. In any case, be wary of any undue pressure to buy a specific product.

Investments

The first step to successful investing is figuring out your financial goals and risk tolerance—either on your own or with the help of a financial professional. Numerous finance-related web sites have quizzes that allow you to assess your tolerance for risk. Once you know what you are saving for, when you will need the money, and how much risk you can tolerate, you can more easily narrow your choices of where to invest funds.

Principles of Investing

Listed as follows are some basic principles of investments:

- Diversification. You should diversify your investments to reduce risk. There are different types of diversification—among companies, among industries (eg, techno-logy, manufacturing, and utilities), and among asset classes (eg, stocks, bonds, and government securities). Diversification affords the investor the greatest protection against business risk, financial risk, and volatility.

- Risk and return. Investments that have the possibility of the highest returns also have the highest risk of loss. Investments that are safe, meaning you will not lose any money, have a lower rate of return. For example, certificates of deposit, which are insured by the federal government, are safer than mutu-al funds; but the guaranteed return rate on a certificate of deposit is lower than the potential return on a mutual fund invest-ment. Money you need over the long term (eg, for retirement) can be invested aggres-sively, whereas money that you will need in the next 2 or 3 years should be invested much more cautiously.

- Liquidity and return. The more liquid an investment is, the lower the possible return. For example, a 5-year bond pays a higher interest rate than a 1-year bond.

TIP

Start investing now; time is the investor's best ally.

Stocks

A stock represents a share in the ownership of an incorporated company. Following are other defi-nitions of terms you are likely to encounter in considering stock investments:

- Growth stocks. The stock of a company that has the potential to increase consistent-ly over a long period is considered a growth stock. The downside of growth stocks is that they often are riskier and more expen-sive than the typical stock. They pay little or nothing in dividends—profits are reinvested in the business.

- Income stocks. Income stocks pay higher-than-average dividends over a sustained period. These above-average dividends tend to be paid by large, established companies with stable earnings. Utilities and telephone company stocks often are classified as income stock.

- Value stocks. A value stock is a stock that currently is selling at a low price; it is out of favor with investors. A value stock is con-sidered to be inexpensive relative to the issu-ing company's actual worth and to similar stocks or the overall market. Companies that have good earnings and growth poten-tial but whose stock prices do not reflect this are considered value companies. Investors who buy value stocks believe that these stocks are only temporarily out of favor and will soon experience great growth.

- Small-cap stocks. These stocks are issued by small companies that have the potential to grow rapidly. However, they are unpre-dictable. Many small-cap companies are rel-atively new, and because of their small size, growth spurts can affect their prices and earnings dramatically. Small-cap stocks are popular among investors who are looking for growth, who do not need current divi-dends, and who can tolerate price volatility. If successful, these investments can generate significant gains.

- Mid-cap stocks. Mid-cap stocks usually are stocks of medium-sized companies. Stocks of many well-known companies that have been in business for decades are mid-cap stocks. Like small caps, these stocks emphasize growth; in contrast, they pay a relatively larger share of their earnings as dividends.

- Large-cap stocks. Stocks of the largest, well-established companies, such as International Business Machines or General Electric, are classified as large-cap stocks. Because of their large size, they are not expected to grow as rapidly as a small-cap company.

Successful mid-cap and small-cap stocks tend to outperform them over time, but large-cap stocks pay relatively more in dividends than do small- and mid-cap stocks. Investors who want their money to remain relatively safe over the long term often are attracted to large-cap stocks.

- Price-to-earnings ratio (P/E). The latest share price is divided by the earnings per share for the company's most recent four quarters. The price-to-earnings ratio is considered a much better indicator of the value of a stock than the market price alone. Theoretically, a stock's price-to-earnings ratio tells you how much investors are willing to pay per dollar of earnings. A stock with a price-to-earnings ratio significantly higher than those of other companies in the same industry suggests the stock may be overpriced; a relatively low price-to-earnings ratio may indicate it is undervalued.

Bonds

Bonds are investments in an entity that agrees to repay the investment on a certain date and make periodic interest payments in the meanwhile. Issuers of bonds can be corporations, federal or state governments, or municipalities. Interest earned on U.S. government and corporate bonds is taxable on your federal return; interest from municipal bonds generally is not taxable.

Bonds are considered safer investments than stocks. Accordingly, the rate of return is typically less than that of stocks. Longer-term bonds tend to pay a higher interest rate.

Bond prices are inversely related to interest rates: the market price of bonds decreases as interest rates increase. If you hold onto a bond until its maturity date, however, you will be repaid the face value (barring a financial disaster).

There are two typical bond options:

1. Call feature. Callable bonds allow the issuer to pay off the bond early. Calling a bond usually is done when interest rates decrease to less than the rate at which the bond was issued. If you hold a bond that is called, you receive the full amount of your original deposit plus any unpaid interest, but you then have to shop for an investment in the lower-interest market.

2. Convertible feature. The investor can convert the bond into stock in the corporation, usually on the basis of a formula specified in the bond sale.

Mutual Funds

A mutual fund pools money from many investors and invests in stocks, bonds, other securities, or some combination of these investments. A fund's net asset value represents the price of one share.

You can earn money from mutual funds in three ways: 1) dividend payments, 2) capital gains distribution, and 3) increased net asset value. Mutual funds are not guaranteed or insured by the Federal Deposit Insurance Corporation or any other government agency, even if you buy through a bank and the fund carries the bank's name.

Most mutual funds fall into one of three main categories:

1. Money market funds. These funds have relatively low risk because by law they can invest only in certain high-quality government securities. Money market funds try to keep their net asset value at $1.00 per share. These funds are highly liquid and often allow you to write drafts on them, like a checking account. Look for a fund that charges minimal fees.

2. Bond funds (also called "fixed income" funds). Bond funds can vary dramatically in their risks and rewards. Because the market value of bonds decreases when interest rates increase, funds that invest in longer-term bonds tend to have more interest-rate risk.

3. Stock funds (also called "equity" funds). Stock funds can increase and decrease quickly (and dramatically) over the short term, but historically stocks have performed better over the long term than other types of investments, including corporate bonds, government bonds, and Treasury securities.

Following are types of stock mutual funds:

- Growth funds focus on stocks with the potential for large capital gains.

- Income funds invest in stocks that pay regular dividends.

- Index funds aim for the same return as a particular market index, such as the S&P 500 Composite Stock Price Index, by investing in all or a sample of the companies included in the index.

- Sector funds invest in a particular industry segment, such as technology or consumer products.

The advantages of investing in mutual funds include:

- Professional management. Professional money managers research and choose the fund's investments.

- Diversification. A mutual fund has built-in diversification because it is spread across a wide range of companies and industries.

- Affordability. Some funds set relatively low dollar amounts for purchases.

- Liquidity. You can redeem your shares at any time.

Some disadvantages of investing in mutual funds include:

- Costs despite negative returns. You must pay sales charges, annual fees, and other expenses regardless of how the fund performs.

- Lack of control. The fund's managers make the decisions—you cannot directly influence which securities are bought or sold or the timing of those trades.

- Price uncertainty. With an individual stock, you can monitor how a stock's price changes from hour to hour, or even second to second. Mutual funds, in contrast, calculate their net asset value at least once every business day,

typically after the major U.S. exchanges close. Thus, you may place an order to buy or sell mutual fund shares, and the price will not be calculated until many hours later.

Following are the most common ways that mutual funds pass on their operating costs to investors:

- Front-end load—a fee that goes to your broker when you purchase shares

- Purchase fee—a fee that is paid to the fund (not the broker)

- Back-end load—a charge when you sell your shares; the amount depends on how long you hold the shares and typically decreases to zero if you hold them long enough

- Account fee—a fee charged to maintain your accounts, often imposed on accounts whose value is less than a certain dollar amount.

Information about a fund's risk, expense ratio, and fees is in the fund's prospectus. It is available from the fund itself or can be obtained from the Security and Exchange Commission's EDGAR database (www.sec.gov/edgar.shtml).

Government Issues (Treasuries)

Government securities are the safest of all investments, but the low risk of a guaranteed investment comes with the downside of a relatively low return. Besides their low risk, treasuries have the advantage of being exempt from state and local taxes, athough they are subject to federal tax. You can buy treasuries through brokerages and financial institutions as well as through the links at the U.S. Department of Treasury web site (www.treasurydirect.gov).

The most common types of government securities include:

- Treasury bills (T-Bills). You buy them for less than their face value and get the full value at maturity—1 year or less from the date they are issued.

- Fixed-rate treasury notes. You pay full face value, and they pay interest at a fixed rate every 6 months until maturity—2, 3, 5, or 10 years out.

- Treasury inflation-indexed securities. These 10-year Treasury notes are offered four times per year at a fixed interest rate plus a second rate that is tied to the Consumer Price Index and is adjusted every 6 months. Payments are made semiannually.

- Zero-coupon treasuries. Notes that are sold at deep discounts below the face value. The longer the term of the note (available for up to 10 years), the deeper the discount.

- Series EE savings bonds (Patriot bonds). These are long-term notes (20 years or more) priced at one half of their face value denomination. They earn 90% of the average yield on 5-year Treasury notes for the preceding 6 months.

Certificates of Deposit

With a certificate of deposit, you invest a sum of money for a fixed period, such as 6 months, 1 year, 5 years, or more. The issuer of the certificate of deposit pays you interest, typically at regular intervals. When you cash in the certificate of deposit, you receive the money you originally invested plus any accrued interest. If you redeem the certificate of deposit before it matures, you usually have to pay an early withdrawal penalty.

Certificates of deposit come in several varieties, including variable-rate and long-term certificates of deposit. Some long-term, high-yield certificates of deposit have "call" features, similar to bonds. The Securities and Exchange Commission web site (www.sec.gov/investor/pubs/certific.htm) has a thorough explanation of how certificates of deposit work and excellent advice for investors.

Annuities

Annuities usually are issued by insurance companies and usually are sold on commission. You invest in the annuity, which guarantees a specified payment or distribution at some future time.

Annuities most often are used for retirement income. You can receive either periodic interest or a lump-sum payment.

There are two basic types of annuities: 1) fixed and 2) variable. With a fixed annuity, the rate of return is set, and the amount of each distribution will not vary over a period as short as 1 year and as long as 10 years. After that time, the issuer can change your interest rate. The rate of return is based on how much you invest and current interest rates, among other factors.

Variable annuities allow you to invest in stocks and bonds, and the distribution fluctuates depending on how your investments perform. If the investments do well, the payment can be higher than it would be with a fixed annuity. The Securities and Exchange Commission has helpful information about variable annuities at www.sec.gov/investor/pubs/varannty.htm.

Protecting Assets

Adequate professional liability insurance has traditionally been the primary means physicians have used to protect their assets, but the ongoing problems in the availability and affordability of liability insurance are changing that picture. Some physicians are seeking ways to ensure their assets are protected in case they can no longer find adequate insurance or in case a huge award exceeds the limits of their insurance.

If a judgment against a physician exceeds the protection of his or her liability insurance, the law provides various ways for the money to be collected. Basically, the assets of the physician may be seized and liquidated to satisfy the judgment awarded. If you want to take action to protect your assets from such a possibility, you must do it before anyone makes or threatens a claim against you.

Property Exempted From Seizure

Certain kinds of property enjoy legal protection from being seized, although the amounts and types of property that are exempt vary from state to state. The following exemptions are among those that apply in some states, with various conditions attached:

- Pension funds in a retirement account, such as an individual retirement account, 401(k), or Keogh plan

- Insurance and annuities

- Social Security payments

- Wages, to a limited extent

- Primary residence, to varying extents

- Assets given away, including gifts to trusts

Use of Trusts

Various types of trust may be used to help protect assets from creditors. Revocable trusts do not offer asset protection, but irrevocable trusts do.

In most states a trust is considered irrevocable unless the settlor (the individual with the assets who initiates the trusts) specifies otherwise. For an irrevocable trust to have asset-protection value, the settlor cannot serve as the sole trustee.

The following types of trusts often are used to protect assets:

- Offshore trusts. Countries such as the Cayman Islands, Cook Islands, Gibraltar, Belize, and Malta have strict secrecy laws and strong asset protection provisions because they do not automatically honor judgments granted outside their own courts. Another important advantage is that the settlor may be the beneficiary of the trust. These trusts must be carefully drafted, often costing $15,000–$25,000 to set up, with annual fees of up to $5,000.

- Spendthrift trusts. To compete with offshore trusts, some states have established this category, which prevents a creditor from obtaining funds from the trust. However, spendthrift trusts do not provide as much protection as offshore trusts.

- Qualified person residence trust (QPRT). This irrevocable trust lets the settlor continue to use a home for a number of years; at

the expiration of that term, the home belongs to the beneficiary.

Other Protection Methods

The following techniques are sometimes used to shield assets:

- Create a business entity, such as a corporation, limited partnership, or limited-liability company, that shields the business's assets from claims of the owners' creditors, and also shields the owners' assets from claims of the business's creditors.

- Create a family limited partnership to protect income-producing assets, such as securities and investment real estate.

- Divide assets with one's spouse, leaving little or no community property. Such an agreement is binding in a divorce, so each spouse must balance the relative risks and rewards of such an arrangement.

- Put property titles in the name of the spouse who has less risk of being sued. This technique would not be useful in community property states.

Sources of Information

- *Financial Planning Handbook for Physicians and Advisors,* by David Marcinko, published by Jones & Bartlett: www.healthadmin.jbpub.com/finance

- *Making the Most of Your Money,* by Jane Bryant Quinn, published by Simon & Schuster: www.amazon.com

Debt Management

- America Saves: www.americasaves.org

- Association of Independent Consumer Credit Counseling Agencies: www.aiccca.org or 800-450-1794

- Bankrate—database and calculators for comparing interest rates on credit cards, mortgages, savings accounts: www.bankrate.com

- Federal Trade Commission advice on credit counselors: www.ftc.gov/bcp/conline/pubs/credit/fiscal.htm
- National Foundation for Credit Counseling: www.nfcc.org or 800-388-2227
- *Pay It Down! From Debt to Wealth on $10 a Day*, by Jean Chatzky, published by Portfolio: www.amazon.com

Loan Consolidation

- Department of Education: www.loanconsolidation.ed.gov
- Collegiate Funding Services: www.cfsloans.com or 888-423-7562
- A primer on loan consolidation, by the Association of American Medical Colleges: www.aamc.org/students/medloans/loanconsolidation/primer.htm

College Investment Funds

- Calculators: www.finaid.org; www.collegeboard.com
- Motley Fool comparison of Section 529 plans and Coverdell ESP: www.fool.com/college/compare.htm
- Section 529 plans: www.savingforcollege.com; www.collegesavings.org
- *Standard & Poor's Guide to Saving and Investing for College*, by David J. Braverman, published by McGraw-Hill: www.amazon.com

Retirement Plans

- Calculators: www.money.cnn.com; www.nasd.com/Investor/Tools/calculators/retirement_calc.asp
- Tax information about retirement plans: www.irs.gov/retirement
- *Twelve Steps to a Carefree Retirement: How to Avoid Pre-Retirement Anxiety Syndrome*, published by the American Medical Association: www.amapress.org or 800-621-8335

- Types of retirement plans: www.napfa.org/index2.htm

Estate Planning

- American Association of Retired Persons estate planning guide: www.aarp.org/estate_planning
- FindLaw for the Public: estate.findlaw.com/estate-planning

Advisors

- American Bar Association: www.abanet.org or (312) 988-5000
- American College of Trust and Estate Counsel: www.actec.org
- American Institute of Certified Public Accountants—lists state societies of certified public accountants that often have referral services: www.aicpa.org/yellow/ypascpa.htm
- Financial Planning Association: www.fpanet.org
- National Association of Personal Financial Advisors: www.napfa.org

Investments

- *The Intelligent Investor*, by Benjamin Graham, published by HarperCollins: www.amazon.com
- *One Up on Wall Street*, by Peter Lynch, published by Simon & Schuster: www.amazon.com
- Risk Tolerance Quizzes: www.rce.rutgers.edu/money/riskquiz/default.asp; www.wellsfargo.com/retirement_tools/risk_tolerance?_requestid=24139; www.moneycentral.msn.com/investor/calcs/n_riskq/main.asp

Stocks

- Bloomberg: www.bloomberg.com
- InvestorGuide.com: www.investorguide.com/stocks.html

Bonds

- Bond Market Association:
  www.investinginbonds.com

Mutual Funds

- Money-market funds information provided
  by iMoneyNet: www.ibcdata.com

- Morningstar—a mutual fund analysis
  company: www.morningstar.com

- Securities and Exchange Commission's
  EDGAR database of all fund prospectuses:
  www.sec.gov/edgar.shtml

Treasuries

- Department of the Treasury's Bureau of the
  Public Debt: www.publicdebt.treas.gov

Annuities

- Securities and Exchange Commission
  information on variable annuities:
  www.sec.gov/investor/pubs/varannty.htm

Index

Note: Page numbers followed by italicized letter *t* indicate tables.